Animal Teachings 2

from Hayley's Angels Methods

Joanne Lefebvre Connolly, DVM

WingSpan Press

Published in the United States and the United Kingdom

by WingSpan Press, Livermore, CA

The WingSpan name, logo and colophon are the trademarks of WingSpan Publishing.

ISBN 978-1-59594-996-7 (pbk.)
ISBN 978-1-59594-970-7 (ebk.)

First edition 2020

Printed in the United States of America
This book is printed on 20% post-consumer, acid free paper

www.wingspanpress.com

Library of Congress Control Number: 2020922948

1 2 3 4 5 6 7 8 9 10

For my 2012 birthday, which came shortly after the completion of my first book, my good friend Diana brought me a present and said: "I have no idea why I'm giving you this but it really wants to be with you. If you don't like it I can return it so no pressure at all." Mystified, I quickly unwrapped what turned out to be a magnificent decorative plate with a very large sea turtle, which appeared to be coming out of it. As we all know by now (please make sure to read my first book "Animal Teachings from Hayley's Angels Methods" prior to reading this one!), life is full of synchronicity (and never coincidences!) explained by the fact that we are ONE, all connected in a web of energies: humans, animals, waters, plants, rocks, planets, galaxies, the whole Universe and the Source. We influence each other for better or for worse. Science has proven that we all are vibrating atoms, therefore we are truly made of star stuff! When we are at our best, we are sharing with the world the best version of ourselves and we create magical ripples that benefit everyone and the whole Universe.

The powerful sea turtle enveloped my whole body and reminded me that it was now time to go home. Home is my shell. Many virtual sea turtles had visited me in the weeks preceding my birthday and I had already received their loving guidance that after giving so much to the world by writing my first book, I needed to now retreat into my shell to re-energize. It was finally time to give to myself. I smiled with satisfaction and looked at Diana with sparkling eyes that said: "Yes, you did it again! Your intuition guided you well and I can't thank you enough for daring to get me this plate! It sure belongs with me, your timing is perfect!" I received the powerful and vivid memory of having lived as a sea turtle in a previous life. I am in fact still living as one today, having kept the same nomadic lifestyle and loner personality. My spiritual feline teacher Bandito went to Heaven at the turn of that same year 2012. He came to me in a dream shortly after his transition into the spirit world and wrapped me in Oneness. He reminded me of who I was, Joanne is pronounced JoONE in French, which is my first language. My current incarnation's purpose is to Be Oneness, Be Greatness!, which became the title of the workshop Bandito & I created together. Here is a message from the Sea Turtles to everyone on the planet:

Always keep swimming, Keep moving forward
Smoothly, One flipper at the time, Slowly but surely
You carry your home with you, Feel safe & retreat regularly
You travel the world, You inspire & Empower others
To Heal & Care for all living beings
To live on Earth as Oneness
x x x x x x x x x x x x x x x x x x x

Thank you Dan, my Sexy hubby, Love of my life, Soulmate & Best friend, for being you.

Thank you to my faithful furry and feathery friends Mocha, Yogi, Sunny, Fuzz, Wilbur, Elvis, Creampuff & Daisy who have been by my side during the writing of this book.

Thank you to my Angels Hayley, Munchie, Snowy, Chicklet, Magic, Bandito, Mister, Cleopatra, Esmeralda, Zen, Chocolate, Velvet, Majestic, Dandelion & Sky for your Heavenly guidance.

Table of Contents

Preface by Michel Pageau

Animals are talking to us, let's listen to them! They hold infinite wisdom and want to share it with us. Their teachings are simple, generous and pure. They teach us, animals and humans, to live in harmony together. They teach us respect and love for nature as well as for each living being we meet. This balance is vital to save our world and help it thrive fully.

Joanne was eight years old when she first visited my wildlife refuge and was sixteen when she joined our team as a guide. Her love for the animals was big, and is still today very inspiring. Her graduation from veterinary school at the University of Montreal in 2001 was a huge celebration and accomplishment that I shared with her as her mentor.

Due to the modernization of our world, we have unfortunately lost the important value of balance that is essential for our planet to flourish and for all living beings to survive. I believe that society's progress has actually made us regress. Most people live life at a reckless speed and forget the essential: respect and compassion for other living beings. Many people "use" animals and natural resources offered so generously by our planet without caring about the harm they cause, or else for selfish, greedy and destructive reasons. They forgot that money is not what is the most important but that human contact and teamwork are. Taking the time to live, share, help and love one another is the right way to live harmoniously together.

I wish that my legacy will be protected and remain alive and vibrant through my great son, Jean-Félix. The flame is burning in his heart. The love and passion for the animals are deeply rooted in his soul. I ask you to help him always remember who he is and help him protect the sacred soul of my Refuge, so the birds can continue to sing, the bees to pollinate, the wolves to howl, the flowers to blossom and the rivers to run. I believe that together we can do it.

We don't come to my Refuge to "see" wild animals. We rather come to receive the messages they have for us. Let's remember that when we see an empty cage or enclosure, there is a beautiful story that accompanies it. It is the celebration of life, of the life of a wild animal who was saved, treated, rehabilitated and freed. That is the mission of my Refuge: helping, loving and caring for animals. We must respect that some animals can't be introduced to the public, which ensures their survival once returned into the wild. These animals thank you from the bottom of their hearts for your understanding and respect. The ones who must stay with us permanently receive as much attention and love as possible. Our goal is to make their life enjoyable and entertaining by playing with them, talking to them and listening to their individual needs. This makes them happy, comfortable and Zen. Charlotte the crow loves to be pet on her neck!

It is with pride and hope that I support Joanne in her life mission of opening the hearts of people of all ages to the rich teachings that animals are offering us. She is a guide to help us reconnect with nature and develop meaningful and profound relations with our friends the animals. Happy awakening to all my friends!

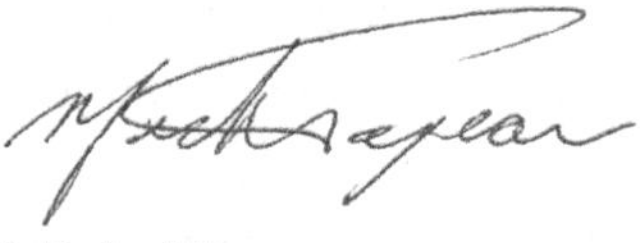

Michel Pageau
Founder of Refuge Pageau
Amos, Québec, Canada
www.refugepageau.ca

Introduction & Acknowledgments

After eleven years spent in the Arizona desert helping over ten thousand families say goodbye to their animal friends, in the comfort of home, our time was up and it had become more than clear. Our lives were being turned upside down. Everywhere we looked, we were being destabilized and uprooted from the life we were used to, but which no longer suited us. We were being pushed away towards greener pastures, literally. From escaping a few too many car accidents to brushing against sticky situations, the message was clear: our Arizona chapter was over and the desert was telling us to leave and find the trees and the water that would make us feel alive again. Above all, it was telling us to not stagnate and become sick in the desert which, although once rich in teachings, was now done teaching us. Amazingly enough, almost overnight, the powerful trees started finding us for real. For no apparent reason, a client gave me a beautiful "tree of life" pendant that she thought I would like, while another gave me a shirt with the same "tree of life".

We had visited California many times over the years, wanting to get closer to the trees and the ocean that we were so attracted to. Understandably, since my husband and I have both lived as ocean creatures in past lives and these memories are still deeply alive and vibrating in our souls and bodies. It became clear that my husband lived as a sea horse since he is mysteriously fascinated by them and has a huge maternal instinct that might be explained by his time as a daddy sea horse giving birth to hundreds of babies. We believe that our dear friend Casey also lived as a sea horse and she is still floating above ground in her human incarnation today. Casey and Dan have a lot in common and truly seem to be made from the same mold. One day, Casey was cleaning out a large office building in the middle of the Arizona desert and found an abandoned sea horse skeleton that she gifted to Dan. Since then, it has become my favorite game to help others awaken those dormant memories, to feel for answers and to remember what bodies they have incarnated in previous lives that may still resonate with them today. I can often see the physical resemblance and personality traits that have carried over from one life to the next, which I will discuss in depth in Chapter 3.

California rejected our presence every time through a series of unfortunate events, such as a flat tire, a flea and tapeworm infestation for our poor canine friend Yogi, a bad foxtail grass encounter for puppy Fuzz, the loss of my husband's wallet, an encounter with a swarm of bees that stung me at a house we were considering buying, a sprained ankle at another potential house, a severe allergic reaction from a plant at a third house, car sickness and the list goes on. Those were thoughtful messages telling us that we did not belong there. Disappointed, we finally accepted that we needed to look at the Atlantic coast of Florida when Casey invited us to go visit her hometown on Amelia Island. That is where we found the perfect property that seemed to have been built for us: a charming nine hundred square foot home on a beautiful three and half acres of lush grass, enchanting old oak trees, vineyard, wild blueberry and blackberry bushes, a private pond and a horse paddock, five minutes from the ocean. It even had "our swing" in the backyard, which seems to follow us wherever we go. We started finding lucky pennies and quarters everywhere on the property and still are finding them more than two years later on this magical land that we call home. I also started seeing my date of birth randomly everywhere. I was indeed reborn.

Having to end my extremely busy veterinary practice in 2016 and "fire myself" was the hardest thing I ever had to do. But since it had pushed my family and I completely out of balance, it had become a life or death situation and the right choice became obvious. Thanks to Chicklet, an orphaned rooster who had taught me "Family First" through our very challenging relationship, I knew that in spite of the intense grieving period that came with closing the Arizona chapter and leaving behind families and their pets that I had been helping for so many years, I had to save my family and myself. I would have to rebuild from scratch in our new home. We do learn most when it hurts, and we also learn most by jumping off the comfortable mountain of achievement we have been climbing for years, once we have reached its peak. Stagnating at the top is a waste of time and potential when there are taller peaks waiting for us to climb. Our evolution must continue throughout our entire life on Earth, and my husband and I have become a powerful team and masters at avoiding stagnation and even speeding up the evolutionary process by finding short cuts to our destination. When our biggest fear became wasting our potential and missing out on life and on opportunities to chase our dreams and live to the fullest, jumping off the cliff became much easier. It actually became magical. That fear gave us wings to dare to live, and nothing could stop us because we had found our path.

This means we have learned to remain open, adaptable, vulnerable, humble and grateful. We have learned to live with our hearts wide open and also fearlessly (or almost), always remaining aware of the signs of guidance, trusting them and the unknown, letting go of control, because we know that when a beautiful chapter ends, another beautiful one begins. It's amazing to see the hidden strengths that we have buried inside of us appear during difficult times of growth and achievement. Our road trip back across country was a little more involved than the first time, having accumulated a lot of necessary material goods over the years. Being so conscious of staying light and only bringing the essential, we still had to face the fact that two large moving trucks would be needed to fit our music, gardening, veterinary and household items. After three days of intense driving with dogs, cats, bunnies and hens, everyone was ecstatic to finally feel the grass under their feet for the first time and meet the Floridian bugs, lizards, ducks, birds, rats and squirrels sharing our new home.

Walking our domain has been a therapy since day one. Enjoying the views, listening to the many birds singing, the wind blowing, feeling the warm sun on our skin, feeling the giant tree roots under our feet, the grass, the sand and the earth between our toes is indeed a therapy that we call grounding or earthing. Grounding with the Earth is becoming oneness with Mother Nature and receiving her life force through direct barefoot contact or through thin-soled shoes. Our horse paddock was empty for only a short time because Majestic begged us to move in. Majestic was the picture perfect horse of my childhood dreams, with a sturdy build and powerful muscles. He was a retired show horse whose living situation had become precarious and who desperately needed a new and better life. We were a match made in heaven. If I had known that Majestic was waiting for me in Florida, I would have had a much easier time moving out of Arizona. This was reinforcement of the importance of trusting the unknown.

Our new life chapter together began quickly and our time spent together was truly magical. How much fun did we have! Majestic made himself at home right away. He cleared and revived the old trail from the barn to the lush pasture and around the pond in which he would regularly cool off and dunk his head to eat pond salad (lush algae and plants growing at the bottom). Another dream had come true when Dandelion and her sisters moved in a few years earlier. Hens make wonderful pets indeed. They love to eat table scraps and they go right to bed when we sing their lullaby. Dandelion did fulfill our dream of having a chicken friend sitting on our shoulder. She seemed to enjoy herself greatly and would jump on us when we least expected it. She also enjoyed going for rides with Majestic, sitting on his plump and cozy butt while he would graze around the yard. We did enjoy spoiling her and her sisters with organic foods of all kinds for many blessed years, and in return, they provided us with the happiest eggs from the happiest chickens.

This Florida life chapter also revived my artistic side by giving me the time and inspiration to create personalized memorial charms made with cremated remains, hair and pictures from loved ones, animals and humans. Hand making simple, meaningful, powerful charms with all my love has brought me such joy, knowing that they will bring connection and strength to the grieving families. They can be worn as a pendant on a chain or on eco-friendly hemp cord, as a bracelet, on a key chain, to hang in our home or car, or can simply be carried in our pocket or put under our pillow.

Once again, I want to thank all the animals on my path as well as their human families. Animals ARE truly the best teachers. I am excited to share this second book with you (printed on recycled paper), drawn from the teachings of the Universe, the Spirit World, Mother Nature and its animals, all of which are continuing to provide me with selfless guidance. I hope I can help you climb the tallest mountains by sharing with you mind-expanding and mind-exploding animal teachings to build a better, more balanced and sustainable world on Earth. Be Oneness, Be Greatness!

Chapter 1

Death penalty explained by crows

In the animal world, "Family first" is a survival imperative. While most animals are non-confrontational and save their energy to survive, they will not hesitate to defend themselves and their family when under attack. A flock of crows will peck an eagle to death for stealing their eggs. Would we call this balance? Everything in the world does need balance. Extremes are rarely good. Karma dictates that you will eventually reap what you sow, good or bad, which is supported by the law of attraction stating that we attract who and what we need to learn our lessons and achieve balance. Synchronicity and signs of guidance always lead us in the direction of balance. Nature teaches balance as well: we need just enough water and just enough heat. Too much or too little of either one causes death.

Chicklet had a very challenging way of sharing this message with me. What a cute messenger he was with the black and white puffy head of a Polish rooster. He was a chick when he came to us, whom we mistakenly thought was a female. The first four months of his life were the most enjoyable. He loved to cuddle and fall asleep on my chest. He enjoyed hanging out indoors and proudly wore the handmade diaper I crafted for him. We were having a blast until puberty hit and he, unfortunately, started humping my head. Talk about a rough reality check. Then crowing began and all my hopes of sharing life with a hen vanished. Chicklet was a rooster.

Establishing boundaries is one of the toughest lessons to learn, but vital to achieve balance. Chicklet needed a family and I needed to protect mine against his physical attacks and invasion of privacy with his loud singing and big personality. That is when we moved the girls in. We rescued a few hens to keep him company, hoping we could achieve peace and harmony for all. He adjusted really well and was very sweet to his girls, impressing them with his daily courtship dance. However, when we visited to clean and pick up the eggs, he became just like the crows and would have pecked us to death if we had let him. Roosters are banned from most cities because of their unsafe behavior. The fact that they crow incessantly at all hours of the day and night doesn't help.

Our living situation deteriorated and became an unacceptable nightmare. Our stress level was at its highest. Reminding myself of the most important principle for survival, "Family first", I had to face the very difficult fact that Chicklet could no longer live with us. We looked at all our options for the best outcome: castration was too dangerous to attempt and finding a farm for him to move to would jeopardize the health of the other birds living at the farm since Chicklet had an incurable and contagious sinusitis, which he had contracted from his hens who had come from a contaminated environment. His daily antibiotics kept him asymptomatic and his quality of life was acceptable, but unfortunately, euthanasia became the only suitable option.

For many days, though I knew what I had to do, I struggled to be at peace within myself with this decision. The day before Chicklet and I parted ways, I received unexpected phone calls from two different women I had helped many months before. They both called to thank me for helping them make the most difficult decision of their lives in choosing euthanasia for their dogs, their best friends, who had attacked another family member viciously. These dogs could not be rehabilitated and would always pose a danger to others. I remembered both of them very well because that type of euthanasia is by far the hardest for me. I felt that the coincidence of them both calling me at this time was the Universe's way of giving me the strength I needed to help send Chicklet to the spirit world. My heart had finally found peace. I knew it was the right decision. I thanked my wise and cute messenger and lovingly escorted him into a better world.

I crafted myself a "Family first" memorial charm made with a feather from Chicklet that I mounted on a hemp bracelet so this one-of-a-kind messenger could travel with me at all times. My physical scars left by Chicklet's attacks would forever remind me of the importance of life balance.

I do believe there is good in every living being. Unfortunately, society has failed many people and animals. Whether it is through abusive relationships, lack of love, lack of proper parental guidance, bad genetic, toxic environment, emotional trauma, society's lack of resources or lack of naturalism, many people and animals become unfit and unsafe to live in our world. I see most of them as souls in distress, lost from their intended life path. One of society's answers to the problem is to keep these people and animals in jail or in an animal shelter to protect others. I applaud animal rescuers who often go through great lengths to rehabilitate animals, even the most aggressive ones. Most animals and people can heal to the extent of finding a safe and dignified place in society for them to live happily with a purpose. I deplore most current prison systems since they appear to worsen the trauma inmates are experiencing as well as increase their aggressive behavior.

A few hopeful and successful prisons in our world are truly showing the way by focusing on rehabilitation. They are not-for-profit establishments and treat inmates as human beings, with respect, compassion, unconditional love, tolerance, understanding and non-judgment. While establishing safe boundaries and a healthy structure for them to develop in, inmates are taught responsibilities and skills to help them re-enter our society. They learn to communicate, express their individual needs, cook, clean, garden, repair cars, play music, exercise and dance, all of which feed the soul and increase self-esteem. Inmates feel good about themselves and feel valued. They get hugged and are told "I love you". They feel that they have a life purpose, a place in the world to contribute to society and that their life matters.

It is important for us all to learn to see others as fragile souls having a human experience and working hard to become decent beings. Every time we catch ourselves judging them for their wrong doings, we must remind ourselves to see their basic goodness and support them on their journey as they try their best to grow within the circle of what they know and what they have. Growing does take time. The more love and support we give them, the easier life becomes for them. By doing so, we become amazing teachers and leaders of the new world we are building.

In the rare instances where people and animals are impossible to rehabilitate and pose a serious threat to the well-being of others, the death penalty, I believe, becomes the most loving and freeing gift. The death penalty becomes a humane and loving euthanasia to free these souls from their tortured minds, their sick and unbalanced mental prisons, which are preventing them from experiencing self-love, growth, compassion, kindness, empowerment and fulfillment. Inspired by the crows, death penalty/euthanasia should be an option we choose to help re-balance society, preserve peace and harmonious living, achieve sustainability and eliminate these sad souls when all other options have failed to guide them, integrate them and help them thrive.

Since Chicklet left the Earthly plane, I have come across wild flocks of hens and roosters living in California and in Florida. I wish Chicklet were born a wild rooster. He would have fit well in that environment and lifestyle. I want to think that he made the decision as a soul to generously find me and give his life to help me grow. I am forever thankful to him for that. This experience led me to think further about how we can prevent souls from becoming lost and distressed in the first place. I believe that the lack of naturalism in modern society inflicts great pain on most animals and humans who suffer without realizing it. Bottom line, our modern society is everything but natural. Society asks us to fit in boxes that all look the same. No wonder so many animals and people behave "badly", feeling completely lost from their essence and stripped from their identity. They suffer from the "pain of existing" and are desperate to find relief.

The most popular option modern society has to deal with this pain is to numb it with antidepressant medication or other buffers. Whether it's a pill, alcohol, cigarette, marijuana, food, television, sex, pornography or any other addictive crutch, it brings a quick fix so one can then pretend all is well instead of facing the real problem and healing it at its core. Younger and younger children are now falling into the same trap. Pet owners and parents request the magic pill to fix their pet's and child's "bad" behavior when the unnatural lifestyle society has created is truly the problem.

We are killing trees and building tall apartment complexes, covering the rich Earth with asphalt and cement that sever our life force and energetic bond with Mother Nature. We all wonder where we belong, where we are going, we feel lost and we don't know why. We continue to breed and breed more children and animals of all kinds who will be as lost as we are because we don't take the time to guide them, we don't know what to teach them because we haven't learned it ourselves, and there are so, so, so many of them that we are completely overwhelmed. These children and young animals end up in shelters, in the streets, and this vicious cycle continues endlessly, until maybe we will decide one day to do something real about it by passing a birth control law that would apply to certain animals and people unfit to breed.

What greater gift is there than to give someone a chance to focus on themselves, to figure out what feeds their soul, to honor their own nature, to achieve self-growth, empowerment and fulfillment? A birth control law would accomplish that. There would be no more accidental pregnancies, which currently represent half of all pregnancies. Parents would be more mature and educated by the time they decide they want a child, if they ever do. Not everyone should breed or be a parent, a concept that elephants understand: elderly females in a herd facilitate mating of the daughters who show the most potential to be good mothers.

Parenting classes would be mandatory in order to adopt or breed animals and humans, and a license would be obtained after completion of the classes. Parents would learn to take care of themselves first, achieve stability and balance, work on perfecting their relationship to be a strong couple and become great teachers. They would then have so much more to give, more wisdom to share, and less children to care for. Life would be better for all.

Violence is escalating because society is not taking care of its citizens and is sadly often harming them further as opposed to helping them. Society must teach its people, not fail them. We are all born clueless, with only our animal instinct to follow, which often guides us into breeding uncontrollably. To make matter worse, modern society has lost its natural selection process for survival of the fittest, therefore the balance is lost and the end result is over-breeding. A healthy society doesn't have homelessness, orphanages or shelters for animals or people.

The earthworms are a great example of population self-regulation, as they slow down their reproduction when space or food becomes limited. Animals can change their reproductive output depending on certain environmental conditions such as population density. Female squirrels shut down reproduction in order to increase their own chance of survival. Having babies is very taxing. The cost of reproduction is extraordinarily high since the mother must provide safety and food for herself and her babies. Only two hundred years ago, humans were like squirrels and reserved breeding for stable and strong couples. Surviving was much harder back then and resources were scarce. The modern world created an abundance of resources and easier survival, and therefore the birth rate skyrocketed. It is now time to remember the animals' guidance and go back to that lifestyle. We can control the chaos and find the new balance for our modern society before we completely destroy the Earth and run out of space, food and other resources.

For as long as I have rescued animals, I have always had the same need to give each of them a more "natural" life. It has always been my priority of achieving this balance because I see how animals respond positively and thrive emotionally and physically. I understand that "life inside four walls" will keep you from getting hit by a car or eaten by an eagle, but as I explained in my first book, there is a fine line between safety and boredom, and we must choose the most appropriate balanced lifestyle for each being in order to prevent illnesses. Cats have an inbred need to hunt. Confining them inside often reduces them to only existing, which causes them a lot of stress and diseases. Even for the prey animals, all the bunnies and chickens that have lived with me share the same opinion on the topic: being outdoors allows them to live life to the fullest and achieve a life of balance. My advice is to listen to each animal and find the most suitable lifestyle for each to thrive and feel empowered, which often results in combining the wild and domestic lifestyles to achieve a balance somewhere between the extremes of safely existing and unsafely living at large.

The same concept applies to children. We must choose the most suitable balanced lifestyle for each one, which always includes spending daily time outdoors "grounding" like nature intended, which helps prevent the soul from becoming lost and distressed. Children and young animals learn by observing and repeating what they see and hear. Teaching them real wisdom and life balance concepts is mandatory. I deplore the violent content, disturbing messages and horrible life lessons of many children books, songs, toys and movies. It is appalling that harsh arcades and video games ask the player to kill a fellow human or hurt the duck to win, instead of using more altruistic activities like picking up garbage, saving animals and feeding the homeless. Children are innately compassionate and caring but we numb and ruin them from the start, and then wonder why they commit suicide at a young age or why they grow up to be so callous, wasteful and disrespectful. Society teaches them to be bad. Moreover, society teaches them to lie.

Some of the most damaging lies causing huge disappointment and mistrust in children are the lie about Santa Claus, as well as the classic love story ending perfectly with "she met Prince Charming, they had many children and lived happily ever after", which sets up young girls for major disappointment later in life. Young girls deeply believe the story and turn into women looking for Prince Charming their whole lives. They experience disappointing relationship after relationship, never finding a partner good enough to be with. Young girls need to be taught that Prince Charming doesn't exist, that we are all a work in progress and that Mr. Perfect is a fantasy. Instead, look for your best friend with whom you can grow old and who shares your love, your values, your passions and your dreams. Animals don't lie to one another. Hopefully we can start telling children the truth and give them better tools, empowering stories and role models to get a great and fair start in life, instead of filling their heads with false and unattainable expectations that may damage them for life. Once again, animals know best. I suggest we follow their guidance and keep it real.

The third limiting belief that I was told over and over

growing up was: "That's normal, that's how life is", which seemed to be the answer for all of my questions and concerns about our world. After years of continuous disappointments and feeling let down by the adults' responses to my questions, I finally had a major breakthrough and told myself in my early twenties: "No it is not normal, that is not how life should be and it is not how I will live mine".

Chapter 2

Wilbur's plea on sexual harassment and prostitution

One early morning as I stepped outside with the dogs, they immediately took off running madly towards our gate a few acres down by the road. I ran behind them as fast as I could, worried about finding out what had alarmed them. To my relief, we came nose to nose with a forty-pound domestic Vietnamese pot-bellied pig on the other side of the fence frantically trying to get in. He was mostly black with a small white star on his forehead, gorgeous highlights in his Mohawk hairstyle and a pink heart on his nose. The frightened creature had a spider web covering his face and seemed completely out of sorts. I decided to bring him in to safety until we could return him to his home.

Of course, this ended up being our home! It didn't take long for Wilbur to make himself so comfortable with us that he turned into a little sex maniac. Within a few hours, he had terrorized all of our animals and ourselves by chasing us, destroying fences and trying to break through our house door to get to us. The story became clear: he was in full puberty just like a teenager, with hormones raging, discovering sex and being completely obsessed by it. He had broken out of his pen somewhere in the neighborhood to find females or any other being he could mate with. Bottom line, no one was going to come looking for a missing pig behaving this way. After reading about pigs' needs and crafting him a "Miss Piggy" from a large pipe covered with soft foam, we sadly remained his favorite attraction. We decided that our only option left was to perform an emergency castration in the hope that by drastically lowering his testosterone level he could shift his focus onto better things and enjoy life with us.

Surgery went well and by the next day, Wilbur had miraculously turned into the best pig. My husband and I were ecstatic and could not believe the drastic change in his behavior. We were thrilled to be able to develop a relationship with him: going for walks with him, teaching him to sit and to walk on a leash, and giving him belly rubs, which he really enjoys. What a smart animal he is! We decided to get him a ramp to climb in the car so we could take him for adventures around town. Wilbur has met people at the beach, students in schools, explored parks and new territories where he always finds different plants and acorns fallen from trees to eat.

Wilbur inspired many ideas about how to help people who have similar issues controlling their sexual urges. Once again, humans are animals. Many humans breed and rape because they follow their animal instinct. There are many solutions to this problem. The first one is to legalize prostitution and sex workers. Unfortunately, society and religion deny that sex is a profound need that if unmet will cause much trouble in society. When humans honor their inner monkey and fill their need for sex, humans become much happier, balanced and able to live better in society. It is true that people crave sex but many people simply crave human contact. Science has proven the powerful benefits of a simple hug, of the human touch, skin to skin, which heals the soul and body on so many levels. The world has never been more populated, yet people have never felt lonelier. Love your fellow human brothers and sisters.

Sex workers would help lonely people heal in a safe and respectful environment. The restrictions of society and religion have created most rapists, pedophiles and sexual predators by forbidding them to fill their deepest animal needs. Yet at the same time, society bombards them with pornography and sexually-based marketing. Suppressing urges can be extremely dangerous and unhealthy. It is completely irrational to think that all men can learn to control or suppress their urges, or think that masturbation is enough, or that hormone therapy is the answer. To the contrary, they need a legal outlet for their hormones. Legalized prostitution is vital and natural. I believe there are enough women with a strong libido who enjoy sex, enjoy caring for someone, sharing intimacy and making friends who would thrive having their own business in this field. With health and safety regulations, they could find fulfillment in teaching society to see sex as a more loving, natural and healing experience.

With artificial intelligence progressing rapidly, society might even benefit from sex robots helping citizens very soon. Look at nature and let animals inspire you. Find your own recipe for happiness. Pick the lifestyle that suits you, to each their own. What works for someone might not work for someone else. Swans, beavers, bald eagles, albatrosses, wolfs, barn owls and gibbons mate for life, whereas gorillas, lions, fruit bats and elephant seals form harems. Many animals will have sexual experiences with many partners and even bisexual relationships for pleasure as well as for social advancement. The goal is to build our relationships based on respect and love in which everyone is happy and free to move on when it no longer suits them. We must be tolerant of one another's differences.

Castration was a miracle for Wilbur and us because within twenty-four hours he became a new being who could enjoy life and not be obsessed with sex. I read a confession from a serial rapist who clearly stated that castration surgery was the best thing that could have happened to him because it freed him from his addiction. There is definitely a place for mandatory castration surgery for people in our society when their hormones are uncontrollably hurting them and others.

The other great benefit of the procedure, or alternatively the sterilization surgery without castration, would be to limit parental failure and protect children. Once again, education means empowerment. Let's do everything we can as a society to set parents up for success, including giving access to affordable contraceptive methods and early stage abortion. The government could offer a monetary incentive to people voluntarily choosing sterilization surgery to avoid becoming a parent. Evolution can unfortunately be a slow process. Just like people who abuse or neglect animals should be punished and denied the right to have anymore animals, parents who have a child removed for cause of abuse or neglect should be denied the right to conceive anymore children. In which case, society should bring as much support and education to help rehabilitate and heal these fellow humans from their underlying problems so the cycle of damaging one's self and others doesn't continue.

Since fifty percent of marriages end up in divorce in America, we desperately need to teach children in schools about philosophy, psychology, sociology, parenting, healthy sexuality and realistic relationships to facilitate communication and understanding of one another. Let's help children figure out as soon as possible who they are and what they need to thrive. Let's learn to see our differences as the strengths they often are that can help us create healthier and stronger relationships. Let's stop judging others, but instead let's help others find and live their own truth and balance in the type of relationships that suit them.

Complacency is a big problem in our world. Feeling like we know enough and do not need to learn anything new, choosing to not discuss difficult topics that deserve our attention, choosing to believe what is convenient as opposed to rigorously and critically thinking whether or not statements or opinions of others make sense. Sadly, too many people believe ignorance is bliss (until it backfires). To the contrary, knowledge saves us a lot of detours, mistakes and pain. We should embrace learning throughout our life. We should not be lazy but challenge ourselves and push ourselves out of our own comfort zone on a daily basis. This builds wonderful skills of all kinds including bravery, resilience and resourcefulness. We should always look at a topic from all angles, even the uncomfortable ones, to come up with the most balanced and fair opinions.

Extremes are rarely good. Nature teaches us balance in everything. Often the answer is: sometimes yes, sometimes no. Unfortunately, our modern society promotes sensationalism where extremes are shocking, good for ratings and therefore money. Agreeing to meet in the middle, to adopt a non-dramatic attitude and to agree to compromise is a boring concept in our modern society. Too many people thrive on hating, belittling and bullying others. We can do so much better. Yes, we can evolve!

Violence in our world would be greatly reduced as well by discussing those same taboo topics in schools. Animals teach us to coexist, to live and let live, to not waste our precious time and energy bullying others but to instead focus on our own growth. If animals fight over resources, females or territory, they do it directly, quickly, simply and honestly. They don't waste time gossiping and telling all their friends about it, or by playing the victim and complaining to everyone around. We should learn to share the Earth and mostly be in competition with ourselves. We should not try to crush others because of fear of others crushing us first, which is a very basic survival reaction. Fear of differences creates division, greed and destruction. Fear of exploring new ways of living impedes evolution. Evolution requires breaking out of the pack, daring to examine his own self, to be motivated to learn, to change and to adapt by taking the best of all lifestyles. Empowering others doesn't weaken us. Learning to work as a team is vital, Mother Nature is clear on that. When we hurt others, we hurt ourselves as we all share the same home, the same land, the same air and the same water. We are stronger together and we need one another to survive.

Animals teach us that zero waste of energy, time and resources ensures survival. Animals don't litter because it attracts predators. Animals preserve their resources and they don't waste them. They only take what they need and leave the rest for tomorrow. They don't destroy or pollute their home. Greedy animals don't survive. Greedy animals eat too much, get fat, get slow and get eaten. Lazy ones get kicked out of the pack or starve to death. Humans must reduce consumption, reuse resources and recycle as much as possible.

Knowing our trash is very important, which is accomplished by looking at what we have thrown into the garbage can. By knowing where the bulk of our debris comes from, we can then stop buying it in the first place. More and more stores all over the world now sell produce and food items with eco-friendly packaging or no packaging at all. We finally had a societal break through by creating dry ball-shaped shampoo and eliminating one more plastic bottle. As discussed in my first book, adopting a vegan diet helps tremendously to save the Earth and the animals, and has shown amazing health benefits.

When animals die of natural causes, they get eaten by other animals or by bugs. I love the Jewish practice of returning the deceased human body naturally and untouched into the ground, which means no embalming, no coffin, no cremation. It definitely is the way nature intended it, to feed the bugs and complete the life cycle. When it comes to my own death, I would like to achieve a natural death in the comfort of the forest where my body serves a last purpose of feeding animals in need of a good meal. It would also fulfill the goal of zero waste.

Zero waste also means involving our Elders in society, like indigenous tribes do, and not waste their precious potential to educate others. Elephants, great apes, dolphins and orcas are some of the animals that look after their Elders as well. Churches should become shelters for homeless animals and humans. Volunteer retirees who desperately want to contribute to society could run these shelters. Shelters for ALL would keep homeless families together: different kind of animals together, spouses together and animals with their owners. We would also match homeless animals with lonely humans and support them in healing physical and emotionally. We would educate, inspire and empower them to re-enter our society stronger together.

Elders have so much to teach to the next generations and it is a waste of their skills, knowledge and wisdom to have them "waiting to die" in retirement homes where most of them are bored, depressed and lonely. It is a real shame to "dispose" of them like they have become useless when they are a precious treasure we must protect, and of which we are an extension. Caring for them until the end is having the honor and privilege to give back to the ones who have given us everything. For the sick ones suffering with no quality of life who have become a "burden", once again, humane euthanasia is a much kinder option than dragging out the agony and dying alone in a nursing home. The way we treat them is how we will be treated since we are tomorrow's Elders.

Animals teach us to live in the present and be balanced each day. Society by contrast encourages us to overwork most of our lives and then to take time to live once retired, if you are lucky enough to make it. People need a purpose at all times during their lives and need to socialize. Since many get sick or die before retirement, it makes sense to live to the fullest and be fulfilled everyday. Zero waste also means to not practice medical torture, as discussed in my first book, and let our dying loved ones die when they are ready and asking for help. By doing so, we save on resources such as time, money, space and most importantly, we don't let our loved ones waste away, suffer and lose their dignity.

Society needs to become fair, with justice for all, which means it must become transparent. The police officers and the court system must become transparent. Police officers need to teach fairness, honesty, balance and peace by example. Just like the animals do, they must preserve their energy for important matters and preserve peace as much as possible. I have met an inspiring flock of roosters in California in which The Sheriff was easy to identify. He was a gorgeous and colorful rooster with a very Zen, yet imposing, attitude. We saw him calmly but clearly stand between the bickering others to restore peace. The other roosters quickly felt his strong energy and showed him respect. The Sheriff was transparent and treated everyone with the equality that they deserved.

Our police officers should use more physical restraint (with martial arts) and depend less on guns to prevent drastic and regretful actions. All humans deserve to get a fair trial, one not based on their skin color or religion but on the crime they committed. Once the judicial system can be trusted, citizens should only have access to basic guns for protection and the most deadly assault weapons should be banned.

Respect of boundaries is important among citizens and the authorities for a healthy society. Unfortunately, most people who commit mass shootings are a product of society, which failed them one way or another. Most people who suffer from true mental illness don't commit crimes. I prefer using the term emotional imbalance to describe the depression, anger and feelings of oppression, frustration, resentment, hopelessness or powerlessness felt by those committing mass shootings. These shootings could have been prevented if society was healthier, kinder and more generous. The quickest way to reduce those shootings is by decreasing temptation. The harder society makes it to obtain a gun, the safer society is. We should require classes in order to obtain a permit, as well as a psychological and personality evaluation. The point is simple: it's like having a chocolate cake sitting on your kitchen counter all day long and trying not to eat it. Decreasing the temptation to wrongfully use guns by making them more difficult to access will save lives.

CHAPTER 3

WHO ARE YOU? BE ONENESS, BE GREATNESS

You are the Source, I am the Source, we are the Source. We are the Stars, the Universe, the planet Earth. We are a group of vibrating atoms. We are energy. We are One with the web of life. The position of the sun, moon, stars and planets at the time of our birth impacts who we are. Each of us is also the total of all his or her combined past lives. For example, in addition to being a French Canadian, descendant of a European ancestor who traveled across the ocean, I embody, remember and channel who I was in my previous incarnations as a Native American woman, a Chinese sex slave, a fisherman raising many children with my devoted wife, a hippie who loved taking hallucinogenic drugs and who fought the injustices of the world, a young boy who drowned in the Caribbean sea, a sheep, a dragonfly, a sea turtle, a wild cat and many others.

How did I discover all of this? I discovered it by getting out of my head and opening my heart. That is truly how messages come, how dormant cellular memories awaken in our body and reveal our identity. Each piece explains a part of who you are today. Are you afraid of water? You might have drowned in a previous life. Are you non-confrontational and just want to turn your back when someone harasses you, shielding with your shell and just wait for the annoyance to go away? You might have lived as a sea turtle.

I have a deep understanding and extreme compassion for others battling addictions that only a past life experience can explain. Remembering this made me understand my current behavior and explained my need to keep all bad habits and routines from forming right away. It is a huge personality trait of mine and I realized how vital it is. I believe that I vowed to experience this current life free from crutches of all kinds, therefore experiencing the raw pain of the world in order to take different and more positive actions to end it. This means I don't allow myself the simplest pleasures (or addictions) of drinking coffee or soda, eating dessert after each meal or any binge eating or show watching. Interestingly, I smoked on rare occasions in college and was puzzled by how natural it felt and how I knew exactly what to do. The experience brought me back to the old days of a past incarnation where it felt so good to numb from the pain of the world for a while, where I could feel the pressure of being, as well as the pressure of dealing with this crazy world, disappear.

Following the same method of opening our heart to let the information flow, it is beneficial to try to figure out the past lives of our animals as well to know them better and to help them fulfill their incarnation. Our dog Fuzz looks like a horse with his mane and tail. I first realized it when, as a pup, he had the habit of sitting between my legs. It gave me the familiar sensation of riding him, like I believe I did in a previous life. He also runs like a horse and has had exercise-induced nose bleeds, which have been reported almost exclusively in horses. The feeling of him having lived as a horse is so real that on a few occasions, other people misspoke asking me about my horse in reference to Fuzz. He is the most loyal friend, always glued to us and never runs away, unless he sees a horse brother, then he runs to him. Our cat Mocha embodies a raccoon with his short legs, puffy coat, raccoon tail and wild behavior. So much so that he even eats his food by grabbing it with his front paws.

Every animal has a life purpose, so pay attention to your pets' likes and dislikes, to what makes them feel alive, and what makes them thrive. Wilbur loves company and loves to explore new horizons. It did not take long to realize how smart Wilbur was and that we needed to keep him entertained in order to prevent boredom. He learned in no time to follow the trail of cheerios cereals up the ramp into my SUV. He also learned that when we put on his body harness it means we are going on an adventure. Wilbur thoroughly enjoys the different smells and tastes of flowers we find in the different parks we take him to.

I was, however, not prepared for the masses of people Wilbur was meant to teach. His soul purpose revealed itself during our first trip to the beach: he is a vegan activist. He is actually the best vegan activist I have ever known. Who better to teach humans that animals have feelings, to respect all life forms and to care for the animals who become their food, than a hundred-pound pig sitting for treats, flopping over for belly rubs and knowing how to express himself with multiple sounds and songs? I realized quickly how changed forever people who meet Wilbur become. Their hearts become open and they experience compassion like never before. They thank Wilbur and then tell me how they will never be able to eat bacon, ham or any type of meat again. Well done, Wilbur!

I find it fascinating how pet owners accurately resemble their favorite animal. There is an amazing attraction uniting us. When I ask people how they have adopted their pets, most of them say that they in fact did not choose their pets, but that their pets chose them. The right animal who is the right teacher for us does seem to appear when we need him or her. Combining this with the fact that we often share physical traits with beings we have lived as in a past life, it makes sense that we attract, and are attracted to, animals that we have incarnated before, and therefore resemble. A friend of mine loves and resembles a Chow Chow on many levels. Another one has a special connection with English bulldogs, another one with Pomeranians, another one with Papillons, and one more with Dobermans. Anyone asked to match them based on their physical resemblance would have no problem getting it right. I have met a handful of reptile lovers and rescuers who shared the tightest bond and understanding with their exotic friends. Some also shared a remarkable physical resemblance with the reptiles they were caring for. This made me think, who better to understand them and care for them than those who have lived as reptiles before? Astonishing.

Think about your favorite animal and write down everything you have in common. Which animal do you look like? Spend some time in front of the mirror. Ask your loved ones for their input. Who do you behave like? Do you think you might know how it feels to have a tail? What did your tail look like? Short or long tail? How fast did it wag? Short or long hair? What color? How about wings? Were they thin, light and colorful like those of a butterfly? Or thick, heavy and feathery like those of an owl? Do you know how it feels to have a beak? Or did you have big canine teeth to bite and chew meat? What did your feet look like? Palmed like those of a duck? Hoofed? Sharp claws? Or maybe no feet at all if you lived as a snake or a fish.

What environment do you thrive in? Are you a winter or summer person, what season do you prefer? Do you prefer the beach or the mountains, water or desert? Where do you feel most alive? Are you a day or night person, Sun or Moon? Are you country or city? Do you prefer noise or silence, nature or buildings? What music speaks to your soul and makes you travel in time?

What is your survival instinct? Fight if you have lived as a predator, or flight if you have lived as a prey? Do you prefer high intensity or low intensity exercise? Do you move or travel a lot? Do you enjoy a nomadic or sedentary lifestyle? What kind of situations do you attract over and over in your life? List ten words to describe who you are (you can ask your loved ones to help you); list five words about your passions and what you love, and pay close attention to how each word makes you feel inside; list five words about what you dislike and pay attention to how those words make you feel; list five skills or strengths that you have; what do you live for in ten words? How do these words make you feel?

When you feel happy, light, empowered, at peace, with your energy flowing and feeling like you can conquer the world, feeling free, like something feels right, feeling powerful and at your best, if it feeds and heals your soul then these feelings equal the RIGHT PATH when making decisions. This is how one should feel at all times. What one word describes you the most? What one word describes your pet the most? What one word describes each of your loved ones the most? Our cat Mocha deeply enjoys music. Our cat Sunny's word is hunting. Play is undeniably the word for Fuzz. Even at eight years of age, he is the eternal puppy, reminding us everyday to enjoy each other's company and take the time to play together. Awaken your and your pets' power and reconnect with your life mission.

Most people have incarnated many different bodies over many past lives so some answers you receive might change as you evolve through different life chapters. The goal is to focus on finding the answers that resonate the strongest now to help you thrive in this current life chapter. For example, I deeply needed the Arizona desert to reconnect with the Source. However, recognizing the end of a chapter is vital to continue thriving. When a situation is no longer beneficial, we must make the necessary changes to find the next best situation for the new and better version of ourselves that we have become. This might mean a new environment, new eating habits, different clothing style, or new work. For me, it meant moving to Florida where there were trees, grass and water.

Each life chapter might resonate more with a particular past life and require us to draw strengths from this one particular past incarnation. Indeed, one animal might be more present in spirit to guide us during a chapter and to awaken the skills we learned when we lived as this animal that will help us today. For other people, their past incarnations and past skills may be blended together and present all at the same time, which allows them to pick what skill to use according to the needs of the situation they face as they navigate through life.

As far as our past incarnations as humans, we may also feel the presence in spirit and energy of our people from those times supporting us today, such as a Native American tribe or European ancestors. Genetics and trans-generational memory cannot explain all the amazing connections and traits I have observed in so many animals and people. Although genes passed on from generations to generations are responsible for many characteristics that make up who we are today, on physical, behavioral and spiritual levels, the differences between family members on those three levels are often huge.

Indeed, everyone has a unique soul purpose as well as different skills and passions that can often only be explained by adding the concept of past lives as different animals and humans. The profound and instant bonds that we develop with strangers confirm the notion of a soul family and energetic connection. When we reunite with an animal or a human with whom we shared a past life, it feels extremely comforting. My husband and I have interestingly experienced many blessed encounters with the souls of departed strangers who seemed to have chosen us to purchase their precious houses and cars because they knew we were going to take the best care of them. By doing so, they freed their mind from all worries linked to the material world and were able to continue their soul journey into the spirit world.

Furthermore, I have met a few people who have a deep sense of having existed on a different planet, who relate to extraterrestrials and who do not feel like Earth is their home. Other people connect with fairies who are the Angels from the spirit world watching over nature and animals, but who also incarnate on Earth to be more involved. These human-fairies love to have fun, let their inner child guide the way, laugh and smile a lot, and would do anything to save nature and the animals. I have also met quite a few wizards who enjoy making magic potions, whether it is in the kitchen with spices or else to heal ailments for themselves and their animals. They look right at home in their concocted chemistry lab that appears to be a continuation of their life in the forest or jungle perhaps as a tribal medicine man or woman.

Once you have answered all the questions listed above for yourself, ask the questions for each of your pets to gain as much insight as possible in order to fulfill each of your pet's needs and honor their nature and identity. I have met a few dogs that genuinely seem to enjoy dressing up and wearing jewelry, like they did when they previously lived as humans. A friend of mine loves to put on fancy vintage dresses and hats like the first class passengers wore during their voyage aboard the Titanic. Interestingly, she is afraid of the deep waters and her name today is France, which supports her strong connection to the famous vessel and to Europe where she feels she has lived in a past life. A very bonded couple visited Europe and remembered their way around a town they visited for the first time, attributing it to having lived there during a past incarnation. I have two French Canadian friends who live today just like they did in their past life together as Native Americans. Back then, they were competing for women and territory. Today, they have neighboring hunting lands and they tolerate each other, but their competitiveness is still present. My good friend Valerie enjoys dressing up, wearing make up and high heels even at home on her days off, which she finds therapeutic. Her sophistication doesn't come from her family who lives very simply in the country, but most likely from the princess she was in a past life.

A lady asked me what animal she had incarnated before. Her facial traits were clearly those of a bird. As soon as I told her, she chuckled and confided that birds were indeed her favorite animal and she listens to them every morning. I could see her as a bird pecking in the field with all her bird friends. Still today, her passion remains to socialize within her community. Another human embodying a bird is my mom. She loves them dearly and her favorite flower is the white dove orchid. My mom most definitely incarnates the white dove's lightness, purity, serenity and elegance. As she grew older and her hair started changing color, a wing-shaped patch of white hair appeared on each side of her head.

One of my dear friends growing up also loved birds immensely. She lived free like one her whole life, loved camping outdoors, discovering the Earth and enjoying nature. Her hair was as black and shiny as a crow. She unfortunately got hurt and suffered from intense and uncontrollable pain, which led her to choose humane euthanasia for herself after three years of agony. She felt like a crow with broken wings, which for her was an unacceptable way to live. She died with dignity surrounded by her loved ones.

I visited a lady-wolf at her home. It was evident that she was uncomfortable with humans and preferred the company of her dogs. She blended right in among her pack of large wolf-like canine companions. Her home looked like the perfect den where everyone felt safe. The second lady-wolf I have had the pleasure to meet, Kassandra, also prefers the company of large canine companions, comes alive at night and prefers dim lighting. Black is her favorite color, she has the personality of a strong, intuitive and protective pack leader, and displays a large wolf tattoo on her forearm. Interestingly, she also deeply relates to the Victorian era of mid to late 1800 with its gorgeous red, blue and purple dresses, which she loves. The Victorian era was also the time of the world's first industrial revolution characterized by progress, ingenuity, poetic expansion, political reform and social change. Specific musical instruments and songs she listens to today bring her right back to her days as a Queen wearing a Victorian-style long dress and long honey-blond hair, walking with passion and devotion down dark corridors while holding a candle in her hand, leading the way for her people and feeling confident, calm and at home. In her current incarnation, she loves to read about romance, witchcraft and black magic, and write poetry inspired by William Shakespeare.

It was love at first sight when she met her husband, who she believes was her guard in a previous life. Ryan truly swims in the same energies, embodying the loyal knight he used to be, from which he kept his very protective, swift, instinctive, guarded and resourceful nature. He is pursuing his passion for blade collecting and sword training and, of course, he was born with the last name of Knight. The iris of his eyes has the same diamond-shaped pattern as his favorite animal, the diamondback rattlesnake, with whom he shares many similar personality traits, in addition to portraying his favorite colors of black, tan and green. Listening to war-style Viking-Nordic music brings him mental images of past lives when he was either charging for battle dressed in a medieval armor, or else hunting in the forest holding an axe, and a bow and arrow. One song in particular gives him the chilling image of his own death from being struck with a spear in the back, and a birthmark is present today in that location. In addition, he has a birthmark on each side of his abdomen, and so does his wife. A different music that makes him travel back in time is the one from Frank Sinatra, which brings him memories of holding a microphone and performing on stage, and also of holding a revolver as a mobster and driving an early 1900 Ford Model 18 V8 car.

The two lady-dolphins I had the pleasure to meet, who live in two opposite places in the world, share the same joyful spirit and bottle-shaped nose. Their inner child is very much alive, they love to laugh and play with their friends.

You might have been a cheetah if you are like my friend

Susan who loves to run everyday. She also enjoys wearing leopard-print shirts, has decorated her house like an African safari, and even her email address includes the word cheetah.

I met Jessica when she lived near the ocean. However, the vast forest of the Midwest was calling her home. She was not thriving on the beach and would often wear her hair up in two ponytails looking like antlers. She feels the safest in the forest among her deer family and has since returned home, where she belongs, to live her best life.

Are you an artist and do you love the sea? The lady-puffer fish I know answers yes to both. She has more aquariums in her home than she can count and she loves to draw. The puffer fish is the artist of the sea. Ely feels more at home in the ocean and although she eats mainly a plant-based diet, seafood is something her body needs to thrive, understandably. I also have a very good friend, Galina, who unmistakably lived as an orca. She is a powerful swimmer and is passionate about saving the ocean. The animal teacher who found her is a black and white cat, her land orca. She is also mainly vegan, but her body needs occasional seafood.

I have met an amazing lady-octopus who walks graciously on Earth but spends all her time in the ocean, and can even weld under water. She is as skilled as an octopus and did live on a boat for a few years. Another sea-creature lady I met many years ago also lived on a boat. Her last name was Sail and she felt more comfortable swimming than walking.

We had a great time figuring out what animal my good friend Karen was embodying. Her favorite activity is to walk along the beaches. She is very social and loves to hang out with friends. I felt that her energy was light like a small creature but very resourceful with skilled “hands”, and so I was looking for an animal with developed paws. Looking at Karen’s hair reminded me of a crab with all the legs on both sides. All the pieces of her identity puzzle were pointing towards the crab as her animal. When I finally mentioned it to her, she lifted her shirt and showed me the crab tattoo on her shoulder that she had for many years. We still laugh about it today and are completely amazed by how powerful this concept of past life is.

Other humans who lived as animals before and have crossed my path include a man-moose, a lady-horse, a lady-donkey, a lady-bear who wishes she could hibernate all winter long, a lady-frog, a lady-border collie, a man-sea turtle and a lady-manatee who have all kept the same physical features and lifestyle. And the list continues to grow.

My husband is an incredibly fascinating human-lion. He roars like one with his powerful singer's voice. He also just recently grew his hair long and we were stunned to realize how much it looks like a lion mane with all its beautiful volume. His zodiac sign is Leo, his survival instinct is to fight (over flight), he comes alive at night, he can see better in the dark then most people and is a little color blind, like the lion. He needs regular high intensity exercise like he did as a lion performing extreme hunts, then he will have long periods of rest. He eats a very healthy diet, mostly organic and vegan, with as little preservatives, processed foods and genetically modified organisms as possible, but his lion body dictates the happy balance he must keep, the kind of fruits, vegetables, nuts and seeds he can eat, with a need for land animal on a regular basis, which for him is chicken. Denise, the lady-lioness I have met, shares many of these characteristics and her zodiac sign is Leo as well.

Astrology is very fascinating on many levels. Since each being is unique but also connected to the web of life as One, it makes sense that the positions of the planets and stars will affect the energy currents and impact one's energy, chakras and well-being on a physical and emotional level. Energy will flow better at certain times during one's life, depending on the individual's identity and birth chart. Astrology can help explain why some people and animals thrive more during a certain time of the year and less during other times.

I often spend time imagining that I'm flying around the cosmos, between planets and stars, to get away from the chaotic Earth and relax in the silent and dark Universe. I find this exercise extremely liberating; it helps me gain focus on my life mission as a human and the purpose of my incarnation. It enhances my connection to the whole Universe, of which I am a part, and enhances my feeling of being Oneness with the web of life. It also brings awareness to the energetic and intuitive wisdom of our heart, a channeling that everyone should be doing at all times in order to sense any guidance coming from nature, the Universe, the animals and our past lives, to live better.

The beauty of this exercise is that we can bring the cosmos into our physical being as opposed to feeling our mind detaching and "leaving" our body to go far into space. Picturing the rest of the cosmos coming to me brings a comforting feeling of being at home with infinite possibilities happening at once for my soul to expand through my physical experience in a human body, while also remaining connected to the Source. This makes us feel like we are everywhere at once, in all different planes of awareness and of realities. This exercise helps us shed any armor and let go of our fears. It allows us to really bring our power to the forefront of who we are, giving us the freedom to be and to take meaningful actions everyday to live our most meaningful life.

Humans who have lived a past life as a sea creature may gain the same benefits from imagining themselves in the deep ocean swimming with the sea turtles, with the whales, crawling on the ocean floor or hiding in coral reefs to get away from the chaotic world above for a while, to relax and to re-energize. Again, we can feel present in our physical body yet protected by being in the deep waters all at once. The brain and soul expansion that reveal themselves is extraordinary as we now feel much lighter in our body, like we are floating or flying with the rest of the

Universe, yet it helps us feel more grounded and able to face our incarnation with much more identity and power.

Many cultures agree on the cycle of the seasons as described below. It makes sense that our life and lifestyle should follow some cycle that will help our body keep its overall balance. Spring = morning, sunrise, beginning of life infancy, new projects and relations. Summer = afternoon, high sun, youth, most active mind and body, long days, eat cooling foods. Fall = evening, sunset, adult phase, slow down, days getting shorter, finish projects, end relationships. Winter = night, low sun, end of life elder, recharge batteries, rest body and mind, eat warming foods.

I do know many people who come alive in the winter and dislike the summer heat, just like others thrive at night when it's dark and must retreat to rest during daylight. Everyone is unique and the goal is to find the unique recipe that works for you, whatever it is. Same thing when it comes to eating. A healthy vegan diet has many benefits as I discussed in my first book. Eating simple foods as nature intended with as little transformation as possible is the goal. Growing our food or obtaining it from local or regional sources are the most sustainable ways. It also makes sense to eat fresh foods available according to the seasons. For some people, including the human-wizards, cooking is very therapeutic. They will spend hours in the kitchen and create magical mixes to delight the taste buds. For me, I prefer to nibble on foods and keep it extremely simple, which means I rarely use any spices, not even salt.

Differences in eating habits among vegans are very fascinating, demonstrating how unique everyone is. For example, some vegans eat a lot of potatoes while others eat mainly raw foods. Both Ayurvedic and Chinese medicine have interesting explanations as to what one should eat based on personality, weaknesses and imbalances. It always takes time to adjust to any new diet and stop craving the old foods. The gastrointestinal tract also needs some time to adjust. Once again, everyone is unique and not one diet will suit all humans. Everyone must follow their intuition and their gut, literally, to figure out what foods are best suited for them. Everything in one's life must resonate with their being and feed mind, body and soul during each life chapter, based on one's unique make up, identity and evolutionary path.

When it comes to food, I am embodying the prey animal I have been in past lives and I am thriving on an herbivore diet. I try to follow the seasons and eat what nature has to offer at different times of the year, as do many indigenous tribes who are genetically built to survive and thrive in specific environments and climates. I do agree that most modern humans from developed countries should aim towards eating a healthy vegan diet for many reasons, including great health benefits. However, many indigenous tribes still thriving today are the living proof of survival of the fittest, and that our genetic adapts to the environment we are in, just like wild animals.

The Inuits living in a freezing cold climate and eating primarily fish produce less fatty acids than other humans to adjust to their large diet intake. Combined with their lifestyle of higher physical activity and lower stress levels than most modern humans, they have found what works for them and perfected it through many generations on a genetic level without developing obesity, diabetes, hypertension, coronary or other diseases commonly seen in our modern society.

Although I accept that some people need meat in their diet, the animals they consume should be given the best life possible and the best death possible, because every living being deserves dignity and compassion, and also because we are what we eat. Stressed, unhappy and abused animals will pass that low vibrating energy to the person who eats them. Animals are best hunted from the wild or from comfortable outdoor living conditions, for the animal's sake and the meat eater's sake. Furthermore, the herbivore animals that will be consumed, like cows, should eat a natural diet of organic grass as opposed to acidic grains sprayed with pesticides under man-made conditions.

The one type of food that no human should ever eat, however, is dairy product. The reason is that humans are not baby cows. Dairy products cause multiple common diseases in humans. Unfortunately, many people suffer from them without ever making the connection, such as chronic constipation, production of thicker mucus and congestion of the airways, as well as chronic inflammatory diseases of the joints and the intestines.

Most people today come from one of two groups of ancestors: the nomadic hunters had a smaller body, were faster, agile and ate more meat, whereas the sedentary gardening tribes had a taller body with big jaws to chew plants. These genetic differences influence their dietary needs today and their ability to thrive or not on certain foods. Unfortunately, the picture has been complicated by the bad genes many people have developed and passed on to their children over the course of many generations, which include food allergies, inflammatory bowel disease, gastroesophageal reflux disease and other digestive issues.

When it comes to animals, the same concepts apply. Wild animals follow their intrinsic nature, just like the Inuits, to dictate what diet, environment and lifestyle are best suited for them. Survival of the fittest applies and only the most adapted individuals breed, therefore giving birth to an even stronger next generation. When it comes to domesticated animals, just like for modern humans, many bad genes are passed down and create diseases. Food allergies (mainly to meat protein) and inflammatory bowel disease are common in our modern pets. The good news is that there are many dogs, and seemingly cats, who do extremely well on a vegan diet. I always find it fascinating when families tell me that their dogs love to eat fruits and veggies.

Many of our cats and dogs have experienced a past life as a herbivore, which is definitely the case for Fuzz, our dog who reminds us of a horse. Indeed, he is allergic to most common meats today but he enjoys his vegan diet as well as sharing my vegan foods. To the contrary of many popular beliefs, most dogs and cats can digest most grains. I actually see many pets who develop chronic diarrhea from popular diets with a high meat content as well as from grain-free diets, which reminds me of astronaut food. It is also so calorie dense that the animals have to eat much less of it to get their nutrition, therefore many pets become quickly overweight as well. They however keep begging for more food because their need to chew has not been fulfilled. Chewing is not only beneficial as the first part of the digestion process but it is extremely beneficial to feed the soul. Spending time eating is very comforting. It relieves stress and is an important need that many animals and people have.

The bottom line is that there is not one diet that fits all, which is true for animals and humans. Both your diet and your pet's diet should be in accordance with your body's needs, soul identity and life purpose. You should eat according to who you are. Listen carefully and feel your way through what's right for you and your pets.

Chapter 4

Intuitive medicine for powerful healing

"A diagnosis is an opportunity to grow, don't make it your identity"

I grew up with terrible horse allergies. Going through my horse rotations in vet school was very challenging. My body kept reacting. My eyes would run, my nose would clog up and drain, I looked like I was crying. Those episodes were unbearable. I have always loved horses and always wanted to adopt one. Horses are truly the most majestic creatures. I could watch them run freely in the fields and graze in the lush pastures all day. A few years ago, as I was having lunch with my mother, we started talking about my allergies to horses. My mom and I always have powerful talks where our hearts lead the way. That time, I saw a movie playing in my head: I was a Native American woman and saw the white men capture our wild horses. I felt deep sadness and had an emotional shock watching my friends running frantically in all directions trying to escape, but in vain. They were captured and taken away to become slaves. I felt so powerless and my heart was shattered. The movie ended and I burst into tears. I was inconsolable while re-living the pain and the profound sadness for a second time. My eyes ran and ran, my nose clogged up and drained for what seemed to be eternity.

That is when I realized that my allergies were actually my body still suffering from the trauma, referred to as cellular memory. Our subconscious mind, our soul and all the cells in our body are impacted by all of our current and past life experiences, good or bad. Our body reacts positively or negatively to these experiences, and our energetic life force either increases or decreases, which leads to emotional and physical imbalances as well as diseases. Unfortunately, but understandably, the conscious mind forgets a lot of these experiences, or might have never even been aware of them when they happened. Since many of those emotionally traumatic life experiences happen in the midst of our busy chaotic modern lifestyle, or else at a very young age before our brain is fully developed, in the womb, or even in previous incarnations, we often don't have access to them.

We should make a daily effort to figure out where an uneasy feeling comes from as soon as we feel it, before we forget about it and bury it in our subconscious mind and cells. Gratefully, by being mindful and searching for answers with our heart, we can awaken our dormant memory from as far back as our first incarnation and even from beyond this physical world. We can bring it into consciousness to process it and heal. By remembering and re-living the trauma I suffered from as a Native American, my body finally grieved the loss of my four-legged companions, found closure and healed. My horse allergies disappeared forever that day.

My good friend Marion had a very interesting experience when she became suddenly afraid of water, to the point of fearing going into the shower, just before her forty-second birthday. She couldn't understand how this unjustified fear appeared out of nowhere until she found help from a psychic friend who revealed that she had drowned in a past life at the age of forty-two. This information made so much sense that it awoke her dormant memory and helped her overcome her fear.

My childhood dream of adopting a horse was always present throughout my life but the timing never seemed to be right. At last, as explained earlier, I was gifted with my dream horse after saving my own life and leaving Arizona. I met one of my new neighbors shortly after we moved into our new Florida home.

The conversation took an unexpected turn when she bluntly asked me: "Are you ready for your horse because I know who he is". What? Wow, talk about timing and synchronicity. "Yes!" I replied with the enthusiasm of a young girl realizing that her dream was finally coming true. Majestic's birth name was M.B. This name resonated on many levels. Majestic Beauty became his new official name, but the sound of M.B. is identical to Aime Be. Aime in French means love. Be in English is to be. How appropriate for this horse to emanate the two most important values of life, love and being. Healing began for both of us. We finally were able for the first time in our lives to just be, to share love and just enjoy being alive. I would spend time with him outside everyday and learned to finally relax. Relaxing allowed amazing feelings of gratitude for our beautiful world, my beautiful new friend and our second chance at life to arise. Needless to say, I never had any allergies to Majestic.

My brain was also finally decompressing. During the last couple of years in Arizona I had, due to my overworked and exhausted brain, begun to fear I had a tumor. My brain felt very tense and under pressure all the time. I was also losing feeling in some of my fingers and my nails had formed deep horizontal ridges. I felt deeply that relaxing my brain was going to be a lifesaver and it was. Gratefully, sensation in my fingers came back to normal after my Majestic therapy.

It is well proven by science that processing our negative emotions quickly, then expressing them and releasing them will allow our vital energy to flow again. When we feel Zen, relaxed and happy, when we feel loved and are hugged, our DNA relaxes, our cells relax, our body releases good and healing hormones, and it activates our DNA to heal our body. When our mind cringes, when we are stressed, our cells and DNA cringe too and cause disease, which alters our DNA, therefore passing on physical and mental diseases as well as fears to the next generation.

Unfortunately, I have met many people who, because of their inability to preserve their life balance, became gravely ill. They have been reminders to me to take it easy and slow down. I met a few different women who suffered strokes at young ages, some who developed chronic debilitating diseases, and a few others who figured out too late how they could have prevented their car accidents. Because of this, I encourage everyone to focus on their life balance everyday.

Once again, why wait until retirement to slow down and enjoy life? Life is now, life is today, there is no time to waste and there is so much to experience. Even fulfilling work that we love, when out of balance, is not healthy. Unfortunately, working until exhaustion will be the demise of too many people. So please save yourself while you can, you deserve it so much. And look for the support of a loving animal companion who wants to join the fight, often sharing the same physical and emotional issues. As it happened with Majestic and I, we find each other to heal together.

Over the couple of years shared with Majestic, he returned to his true nature given to him by the Source. He grew his beautiful wild mane back, he returned to being independent, strong, self-confident and wild. However, he would have followed us to the moon to get a taste of those delicious watermelon popsicles we made to cool him off. We would save the rinds, cut them in pieces and freeze them. What a treat! Because Majestic was an old guy, his arthritis finally caught up with him and he developed chronic pain in his feet. We kept him comfortable with pain medication for quite a while, while continuing to soak up all the love and happiness he had to share with us. He did really well for a long time.

Then one night, I had a powerful and celestial dream that I will always remember. Majestic had angelic glowing white fur with long and powerful wings. I had my arms wrapped around his strong neck and we were flying together in Heaven forever!

We were both having the best time, we were finally Home, happy, ageless and free! The next morning when I woke up, I found Majestic in the worst pain. I was heartbroken but I knew that he was finally ready to go Home. I felt really blessed that he had visited me in my dream to make it clear that the time had come. I found the peace and the strength needed to honor his wishes and help him transition into the next world.

Here are a few animal and human stories showing how intuitive medicine for the mind, body and soul can help heal and minimize suffering.

1. Chewy

Chewy was a feline patient of mine who visited her mom in a dream to give her a very important message. She was nearing twenty years old and was mom's best friend. Her frail body was riddled with arthritis but she did not seem to want to let go. Then one afternoon, Chewy had a slight seizure and mom called me. I went to their home and helped mom make the decision to help Chewy transition into the next world. Later that day, mom remembered a dream she had a few days before and it brought her so much peace and closure because it was clearly Chewy's way of telling her that her time had finally come and that everything was going to be ok. The dream started with mom in an old train depot. The depot had no other humans in it but was full of cats lounging on the benches, under the benches and on window-sills. Everyone was quietly grooming themselves and each other. Mom was looking and calling frantically for Chewy. She sat down and suddenly saw Chewy next to her. She sat quietly with mom as they looked around the room together. Suddenly, mom heard the train whistle. She got up, walked out on the platform to board the train and saw a big old steam locomotive approaching. Mom wondered who the train was going to pick up because there were no people present. The train slowed to a crawl and mom went back inside the depot to find it empty, no Chewy or any of the other cats. Puzzled, she went back outside and the train was gone. Mom believes all those cats were there to help Chewy and one another board the train for their journey to cross to another world.

2. Sailor Moon

Sailor Moon was a ten-year-old Australian Shepherd battling acute renal failure. Her mom is a close friend and colleague of mine. Mom called me in extreme distress because she had hospitalized Sailor Moon and for several days had already aggressively treated her with all the medications conventional medicine had to offer. Unfortunately, her kidney values were extremely high and she was dying. Mom was stressed to the max and kept repeating: "She can't die, she can't die, it can't happen, I can't lose her, I'll die too". Facing such a critical situation, I knew we had limited time to shift the energy into a healing one if we had any chance at all to save her. I told mom straight out: "You must make peace with the fact that she might die. Our only chance at saving her is if you stop forcing things because she will die just to teach you that you don't have control over everything". As impossibly difficult as it was, mom had the most powerful talk with her beloved girl, telling her how much she wanted her to stay but that she was giving her permission to follow her destiny, and that she was going to be ok with her decision. Mom realized how good their life was before she got sick, and that all we need in life is love and to go for rides in the RV with our four-legged friends. Happiness is simple and there is no good reason to ever worry or complain. Amazingly enough, because of this new awareness and because mom was able to let her go and surrender to higher forces, for the greater good, the energies shifted and Sailor Moon made a miraculous and complete recovery in just a few days. She lived another four years and had a great quality of life. She died of old age with normal kidney values. Mom grew so much through this experience. Sailor Moon taught us that once again, we attract diseases and obstacles to grow and become more balanced beings and that once the life lesson is learned the disease and obstacle go away.

3. Precious

Precious was brought to me at the hospital. She was an eight-year-old tiny Chihuahua. I was the third veterinarian to try to help her. She was critically ill with inflammatory bowel disease. Her condition was so severe that she was losing proteins through her bowels and near the point of no return. When I told mom that our only chance at saving her was to start her on Prednisone right away, mom was adamantly refusing: "I hate Prednisone, it's evil". What better famous last words to attract her dog's illness and teach mom an important lesson. Obviously, Prednisone would be the only medication able to save Precious's life. Despite her rigidity, mom allowed me to communicate with Precious to see what she thought of the situation. Precious clearly communicated to me that she wanted to live. I begged mom to give her a chance at life. Mom was able to swallow her pride, follow my recommendation and help Precious make a miraculous recovery. Patients with the same disease often must stay on Prednisone for very long periods, if not forever. Thanks to the amazing shift in mom's energy and attitude, Precious was off Prednisone six months later and continued to do well.

4. Jewel

Jewel was a six-month-old Miniature Pinscher puppy just rescued from the shelter. She was really scared when I met her. She had just been spayed and was prescribed antibiotics for infectious tracheobronchitis. Her new owner had to force her to take her medications, which scared her even more. She was now hiding, refusing to eat and my colleague had recommended giving her fluids under her skin with a needle to prevent dehydration. By the time I examined her, her spirit was broken, she had shut down and was ready to die. Mom thought it was time to euthanize her. Jewel looked good physically with no trouble breathing and no nasal or ocular discharge so I asked mom if she was still coughing, mom said no. I then suggested that we stopped scaring her with the antibiotics and that we focused on only giving her love, which meant no fluids under her skin, not forcing her to eat, no abrupt handling of any kind. We agreed that doing less was our best chance at helping this little cutie heal from her emotional trauma and learn to trust people. Thankfully, Jewel decided to live. She improved everyday and is still healthy and happy five years later.

5. Bandito & Mister

Bandito, our amazing hospital cat who was almost twenty years old, and I had become very close. We would take our lunches together. Bandito was determined to teach me balance by gently but forcefully biting me when my brain was on overdrive, overworking and planning my following week's schedule during my lunch hour, instead of relaxing and being in the now with him. I was worried about leaving him to take a three-week vacation I had planned and told Bandito that I really wished he would wait for me to return so I can be with him for his transition into the next world. I went over the calendar days showing him when I was leaving and when I was returning. On my last day at the hospital before leaving, Bandito chose to follow me everywhere all day long. Everyone noticed how unusual his behavior was and I felt reassured that he was going to wait for me. Indeed, he did and we spent many more months together.

Then the year ended. Every employee took well-deserved staggered vacation time to enjoy the holidays. On the first day when all employees were back together at the hospital, Bandito was waiting to share his most amazing gift with us. When we arrived at the hospital, we found him not wanting to get out of bed. His body temperature had dropped significantly and he was dying. The whole team got the opportunity to discuss his care, everyone was able to express how they felt and what they thought was best for him. Everyone listened, showing patience and understanding towards one another's feelings. Finally, everyone agreed to facilitate his transition with medications. If our world's leaders could only be humans as good as our small hospital team, there would be peace on Earth and no suffering. Bandito left his earthly body extremely peacefully and feeling loved. He left us with the amazing gift of Oneness, which means being interconnected as One with all other living beings. Bandito taught me this word shortly after his passing. I had never heard of it until then.

Mister was the other hospital kitty. He had a difficult time following the departure of Bandito and disturbingly lost a few pounds. Mister used to join Bandito and I during our lunches. I was missing Bandito and had stopped going to the lunchroom to eat. Our routine had changed and I realized how much it had affected Mister. I began paying extra attention to Mister and re-established our routine, which brought Mister back to life. His appetite returned to normal and he gained all his weight back.

6. Lexi

Lexi was a middle-aged dog living the good life and spending lots of times outside until a bat bit her. Sadly, she was forced into quarantine at the hospital for three months. We all felt terrible for her. The stress of being confined to a small kennel indoors made her age more during that time than she had in her seven years of life. In three months, her coat had turned shockingly grey. Science has proven indeed that stress speeds up the aging process and oxidation of the cells. Luckily, our daily communication sessions and pep talks helped to keep her healthy and she was able to return to her good old life. Five years later, she is still spoiled, happy, free and enjoying life to the fullest! Go Lexi!

7. Cleopatra

I came home one day feeling extremely overwhelmed and angry at the world's overpopulation problem. I wanted to tell every human and every pet owner to stop breeding, now! Knowing how impossible that was to accomplish and seeing so many homeless animals in the streets and in the shelters filled me with pain and a feeling of powerlessness that was very difficult to process for a veterinarian like me. I have a strong maternal instinct and want to save them all. I was very surprised by how strong those feelings actually were, how much I cared and how hard it was to let go.

Cleo, one of my hens, decided to help me with the process. She started laying her eggs in a different and more difficult spot for me to collect every morning. Furthermore, she sat on them all day long and would peck to make me bleed if I tried to take them. I quickly realized the trouble I had gotten myself into by having radical and unbalanced thoughts about breeding. Since Chicklet was with us at the time, the eggs were fertilized and could hatch into about two dozens of chicks! Cleo made me swallow my words and forced me to accept the fact that breeding was necessary for survival of the species by sitting on her eggs for a good two weeks. Everyday I got to make peace with the fact that I might become the proud pet owner of twenty something more chickens… what a tough lesson. I did beg Cleo to let go of her eggs, I assured her I had learned the lesson and thanked her for the opportunity to grow. Thankfully, she finally decided that I had repented enough. She abandoned her eggs and I was able to prevent them from hatching.

8. Sunny

Sunny joined our family within a few minutes of birth when a Good Samaritan brought him to the hospital where I worked. He was the tiniest kitten with his placenta still attached. We suspect that his wild mom had to escape predators and left him behind. My husband and I gave him a chance at life and started bottle-feeding him around the clock. It did not take long for Sunny to turn into a mighty predator, hunting us inside the house when he was only a few months old. He would have been a great wild cat. He was so intense that we rescued another kitten as a playmate, but also to spare our legs and arms from his attacks. We also trained him to wear a harness to go outside so he could be more emotionally balanced and fulfilled. We trained him to sleep in at night for safety, but we finally had to compromise and give him his full freedom during the day by letting him be unharnessed outside. Being outside brings him so much joy that the few times we forced him indoors for more than a day or two, he became constipated and we had to medicate him. It made complete sense that his body would become blocked, like his energy and his mind. He is now fourteen years old and is doing wonderfully well, keeping the balance between safety and fulfillment by enjoying his daily adventures outdoors.

9. Moustache

Moustache the cat lived with my grandparents who were reluctant to let him roam the yard and would only allow him outside on a leash tied up to the door. Consequently, Moustache suffered through a few too many painful urinary blockages when his bladder would fill to the max and he could not urinate. He was prescribed a special food and also medication for his newly developed diabetes. When both my grandparents died, my mother adopted Moustache. She deeply empathized with his frustration of not being allowed to roam his territory outside all those years, and therefore freed him. Moustache embraced his new kingdom and came back to life. He was finally able to live life to the fullest, to feel the grass and explore the world without limitation. His body responded amazing well to this new life force and began healing. Within a few years, he became the healthiest and no longer needed the special food or medication.

10. Amy

Amy was an eight-year-old Maltese. She was unfortunately grabbed by a large dog who had torn her abdominal wall on her side near her back. Luckily, her skin had been preserved but her organs had herniated just under her skin. She needed emergency surgery to push her organs back in and repair the tear. The specialist was recommending that I make an incision not only over her hernia, but also over her belly near her belly button to have full access to her whole abdomen and inspect all of her organs to make sure there was no other tear or leak needing to be repaired.

But Amy was telling me otherwise. I was extremely conflicted while preparing for the long procedure. When the time came to make the incision over her belly button, I just could not do it. I could not bring myself to pierce her skin. Amy's tiny size made maintaining her body temperature within the normal range challenging while under anesthesia and at the last minute, I cringed as I felt my body tie in a knot. A movie appeared in my head showing me our patient dying because we were doing too much. I knew what I had to do. I told my loyal nurse to re-position our patient into the position I felt made more sense for me to repair her hernia in as little time as possible. I knew it would limit my ability to explore her whole abdominal cavity from that angle but I could still peak and notice any obvious leakage that would warrant a more in depth exploration.

Remembering Amy's vitality when she came in, her alert behavior was telling me that trauma to major organs was unlikely. For the most part, life is a series of guesses where we try our best to make the right decisions but risks are always present. Now once again, no option gave me the guarantee that my patient would survive. I followed my intuition, my heart, my gut, my inner voice and the flow of energy, which have always been my best guides. Most importantly, I listened to my patient and she made a quick and full recovery.

11. Yogi

Our sweet little boy found my husband and I just a few months following Hayley's transition into the next world. We were both still grieving deeply and were not sure if our hearts were ready to welcome another dog. It didn't take us long, however, to realize that Yogi fit in our family beautifully so the timing was perfect. Yogi had a long and full life, filled with exciting road trips, hikes, canoe and kayak rides. He was easy to carry around, loved to ride on our lap in the car and would sit quietly in the shopping kart at the pet store, with a human look and lip that no one could resist. Yogi was a feisty little Schipperke and Chihuahua mix, patrolling the borders of our property daily to keep us safe. He would sleep deep under the covers at night and kept us entertained with his agility tricks.

He was healthy his entire life and never needed any medical or dental procedure, thanks to our weekly teeth-brushing routine at home. He aged gracefully and, thankfully, made it well into his senior years. Then one day we found him in acute and severe pain, with one of his eye severely swollen. There were also multiple painful sores all over his back draining fluid. Only valley fever could explain his symptoms, which he had been exposed to in Arizona, but he had not developed symptoms until his old immune system became too weak. We knew he was in a critical situation. While waiting for my husband to come home later that day, I gave Yogi the strongest pain medications possible but also got his euthanasia medications ready.

Reminding ourselves that suffering is much worse than dying, our goal was to be fair to him. We did tell him that it was up to him to stay for however long he wanted. We gave him the permission to follow his journey and not sacrifice himself for us. Yogi miraculously responded quickly to the pain medications and returned to having a great quality of life. We started giving him the valley fever medication, which took a good month to heal his eye and skin. We were so happy to get this extra time with him. He gave us four more months of total bliss and pleasure, taking his long walks around the property again, greeting us, rolling in the grass and going for car rides. We were so amazed by his complete turn around and felt extremely blessed.

Finally, the time came when he stopped eating, refused to take his medications and stopped going for his walks. His journey on Earth was completed. He took his last nap in the sun, during which we escorted him into the next world with dignity and love. Well done, Yogi, and thank you for everything, from the bottom of our hearts.

It is very difficult to watch nature takes its course, even under the best of circumstances. We feel so powerless watching our loved ones get old, become frail and vulnerable, even if it is how nature intended it. We are extremely grateful to have had the privilege of watching Yogi live a long and full life. We also are extremely grateful we were able to free him with euthanasia. Death is inevitable. Death with dignity is a gift. Watching my little boy pass so peacefully, without pain and while feeling so loved, I can only wish, once again, that every animal and human would receive such merciful help to transition into the next world when they need it.

12. Angel

Angel was a two-year-old cat who ate a long piece of thread and had been vomiting intensely for two days. The string was very long, caught under her tongue and reached down her stomach into her intestines that were bunched together. She was very sick. Surgery was the best option to remove the string completely and save her life. Mom and dad were young, had other rescued animals and did not have the funds to have the surgery performed.

Mom and dad had made the sad decision to free her from her suffering with euthanasia. When I met Angel, I sensed that it was not her time to leave her body yet. I felt the strong bond that she had with her humans and her unconditional love for them, which felt like a mother's love. Her humans were genuinely good, caring and compassionate human beings. They were devastated by the thought of having to say goodbye to her.

That's when I had a possibly life-saving idea. My body filled with adrenaline and I sprung into action. After receiving mom and dad's blessings, we sedated Angel and I grabbed the string caught under her tongue. We pulled and pulled and pulled until it snapped. We removed about two feet of string. Her intestines still felt bunched up so we massaged them while our patient was waking up. The whole staff gathered around her, everyone united to infuse her body with as much love and healing energy as we could.

The next day, Angel started eating. She passed the rest of the string in her stools and healed completely.

13. Bosco

Bosco was a three-month-old Pitbull puppy full of life. The world was his playground and everyday was filled with over-the-top joy and fun! Playing is fun until someone gets hurt. Indeed, Bosco fractured and severely displaced both bones in one of his front legs. Surgery was highly recommended by specialists as the best option for maximum healing. Because his mom and dad were not able to keep Bosco calm and restrict his activity, I had high concerns that performing surgery would lead to complications and bone infection.

My common sense was telling me that since Bosco was actively growing and producing new bone cells at a rapid rate, all his body should need was a little help aligning the bones and stabilizing them, which could be done by gentle manipulations under sedation and avoid invasive surgery involving cutting his skin, exposing the bones and securing them with orthopedic hardware.

Bosco's family chose the conservative option. We followed up with Bosco almost every week. Bosco would come in for bandage changes and more often than not, his bandage was a wreck, dirty with weakened support from the lack of supervision from his family and excessive exercise. Bosco, however, made a rapid and full recovery nevertheless. His young and vibrant body was able to heal with minimal intervention. Common sense always wins.

14. Max

When Marsha rescued Max from the shelter, she had no idea the journey that she was embarking on, but she sure had picked her perfect teacher. Max, an anxious, fearful and aggressive Poodle, came into her life to help her learn the very difficult lesson of setting limits for herself in all aspects of her life. Marsha is one of the sweetest people I know. She loves to please everyone around her but she would often forget to respect her own boundaries. Living up to his name, Max pushed her to the maximum limits. Even though she thought of giving up multiple times, she was determined to make her new relationship with Max work; to gain his respect and to teach him love and trust. Five years later, life is grand. Marsha learned to be assertive and Max learned to listen and respect her boundaries. Both Marsha and Max have become the most balanced and best versions of themselves for harmonious living. I could not be more proud of them. Long live Marsha and Max!

15. Jana

Jana was a young woman when I met her about ten years ago through our love for horses. She grew up with them and was on her way to becoming an equine veterinary dentist. From a very young age, she had been a female in a male industry and had to constantly prove herself and fight for her place and credibility. In other words, for years, she spent tremendous amount of life energy marking her territory. Her body had followed by developing urinary tract infections on a monthly basis. As she finally became more confident in her skills, more comfortable with the great person she was and started receiving the recognition that she deserved, the need to mark her territory disappeared and so did her bladder infections.

In addition, she also battled an extremely acidic sweat to the point of bleaching her shirts. Jana recognized how hard on herself and what a perfectionist she was. She realized that her body needed more sweetness and gentleness. Jana learned to praise herself for her achievements and hug herself after giving her best effort, even if perfection was not always reached. She learned to not criticize herself so harshly and to show herself love, compassion and tenderness. Her body followed her mental shift and she found balance. She is no longer damaging her shirts.

Chapter 5

Do animals commit suicide?

Fuzz is a gorgeous red merle Australian Shepherd that we found in the streets when he was a puppy. He has always had so much energy that he could generate electricity for a whole town if we had a way to convert it. Our other dog, a Chihuahua mix named Yogi, had been the king of the house for five years when Fuzz showed up. Adopting a new animal is always a risk, as the dynamic will change for better or worse. Yogi's feelings were very hurt at first and we were afraid he might commit suicide. I have encountered multiple animals that did commit suicide during the course of my career, meaning that they took an exit door when they disliked a situation.

If you are not familiar with the concept of exit doors, please read about it in my first book. Obviously, suicide happens in people too. Everyone is familiar with people intentionally ending their lives with a gun or overdose of medications. The type of suicide that I will focus on here is, however, a different kind of suicide that occurs in both animals and people. It is one that is unintentional and happens on a subconscious level via what looks like an accident or a disease.

What is common to all types of suicides, however, is the feeling of wanting to escape a situation that seems unacceptable and insurmountable, when the person or animal believes the only option is to die. Again, it never has to be conscious. For example, a toxic and unbearable relationship will cause illness and death to one of the spouses when divorce would have been a better option to escape and find happiness. A cat was killed by a hawk just when his family was relocating to a new house. Another couple divorced and as mom was moving out, on her birthday, her favorite dog ran in front of a car and died. A few days before we moved into our new home, we found one of our hens had passed away.

An animal may chew through a bottle of medications and overdose when feeling that he no longer has his place. A colleague of mine's old horse suffered from colic and died as soon as she retired him from competition and adopted a younger horse. We knew an exit door presented itself to Yogi when Fuzz joined our family, and we worked hard to make sure he chose to continue the journey with us. With much gratitude, Yogi overcame the challenge of sharing his territory and we keep doing our best to make him feel special every day, even seven years later.

Just a couple of years ago, it became Fuzz's turn to reach an exit door. My husband and I were going through some unbalanced times, juggling too many things and feeling overwhelmed when Fuzz swallowed pieces of a toy. This behavior was very alarming and completely out of character for Fuzz. It was the sign that prompted us to re-balance everything in our lives. We made sure to reassure Fuzz that he had his place with us and, luckily, he agreed to stay, did not get sick and never swallowed another toy.

As discussed in my first book, we will all die by choosing an exit door at some point, sooner or later. Therefore, choosing an exit door is not necessarily a wrong decision, but it is all about timing and choosing the right one. My best advice is to make sure that you and your loved ones, animals and people, are satisfied with your lives, share as many years together as possible, overcome many challenges, continue to grow together, and then take the most appropriate exit door.

I have met quite a few pet owners not wanting to talk about euthanasia in the presence of their pets or even in their absence if the time was not right. They felt like they were going to jinx themselves if they pronounced the words. They also feared that their pets would perceive that shift of energy and possibly feel rejected and let themselves die prematurely by taking an exit door when the time was not yet right for them to leave. I have caught myself doing this too and, therefore, I fully support others in following their feelings to pick the right time and place to have the conversation, with or without their pet.

When one of our loved ones reaches the right exit door, it is very helpful to give that animal or person permission to die, as well as space. Most people become upset if their loved one dies during that two-minute break they were away from them. Giving another being space facilitates the dying process and makes it easier to break those amazingly strong energetic ties and love bond. It is simply easier to die naturally when alone so one can focus on himself solely and not worry about the loved ones he leaves behind.

We pampered our last hen, Daisy, to the fullest by letting her sleep with us in the house and hang out with us in the sunroom, which literally turned into her coop for one year. Daisy had a blast. She would still wander the yard and eat bugs for short periods but her arthritis kept her close to home. She hung out with us while we ate and we shared with her our leftover tomatoes and melons, which she particularly enjoyed.

On her last day, she could no longer get out of her comfortable doggy bed. I knew the time was near but I could not bring myself to euthanize her. I deeply felt that she could transition on her own. I sat next to her and begged her with all my heart to free herself and go be with her sisters waiting for her in Heaven. She was safe, comfortable and was not suffering so I gave her time and space to let go. As discussed in my first book, when the patient is suffering, animal or human, euthanasia becomes the best decision to end suffering, and I then encourage the whole family to be present to comfort their dying loved one. When I came back to check on Daisy less than twenty minutes later, she had already transitioned into the next world. Thank you, Daisy, and well done!

Another powerful transition into the next world was the one of Kona, a German Shepherd who had battled severe aggression issues towards people and animals since he was a puppy. I shared the beginning of his story in my first book, and I could not be happier to now share that he overcame his fears and did become the well-balanced leader that he was born to be. Unexpectedly, at seven years of age, after having the best time socializing with everyone at a family party reuniting over thirty people and many animals, mom found Kona resting in his favorite bed where he had just passed. You are amazing Kona, life mission accomplished!

I also find it very important to give permission and space for the soul to fully leave the Earth plane and not become earthbound. Our loved one's soul must follow its journey into the spirit world and may or may not always be able to watch over us. When Bandito died, I strongly felt his presence for a couple of weeks as he was surrounding me with a divine boost of inspiration to create our workshop. As soon as I completed the task, I felt his spirit leave and I burst into tears, finally grieving his loss.

A similar experience happened to my mother-in-law when she had to say goodbye to her beloved kitty Figaro. She strongly felt his presence for a few days following his euthanasia until she told him: "It's ok Figaro, you can go now, I'll be ok". She immediately felt his spirit leave, which brought her peace, closure and the ability to move on into her next life chapter. Knowing that many of our loved ones will reincarnate and find us again, with much gratitude for our time shared, we must indeed free them to follow their soul plan while being hopeful that they will communicate with us and send us signs from the other side if they can, and that our paths will cross again, in Heaven or on Earth. Quite a few families have shared with me how their departed pets also seemed to visit by borrowing another animal's body, either a housemate or a wild animal, as they noticed in that animal a sudden and temporary change in behavior, interaction or even in smell, reminding them of their departed pet.

I believe this happened when a gorgeous western shovel-nosed snake came to witness Sophie's peaceful transition into the next world and home burial ceremony. It appeared in the garden, where her family had never seen a snake like it in all the years they had lived there, and it did not leave for a good twenty minutes. There was something unusual about its presence, as it seemed to be the messenger telling Sophie's family that she had arrived safely in Heaven and that it was ok to let her go.

Three weeks after my mother's cat, Pacha, made his transition into the spirit world, he gently clawed her cheek like he had done a few times to wake her up when he was alive. He left a mark and even made her cheek bleed from the spirit world, saying hello and letting her know he was thinking about her. Squishy also visited from heaven multiple times over many years. His family would hear him run in his hamster wheel during the night, and roll on the floor and hit the walls in his hamster ball that he loved so much during the day. Daisy was only a teenager when she left our world in a car accident. She made daisy flowers grow in her mom's backyard in the middle of the winter from Heaven. After the leader of the pack passed away, mom realized that she could calm down the five remaining canine housemates by putting Baron's urn filled with his cremains on the floor in the middle of the living room when there was a tussle, and then everyone would settle down, just like when he was alive.

Joey's mom and I witnessed the most magnificent miracle when her feline best friend and love of her life, Joey, came back to find her again. I had just helped Joey pass peacefully in the comfort of home and mom was completely devastated, feeling like she had lost her only child. Shortly after his passing, he visited mom in a dream in which he woke her up like he used to do, by purring and rubbing against her face on both sides, then jumping down on the floor. The dream was so vivid and the noise of jumping down was so loud that mom woke up for real. When she looked at the clock, it was the same time at which Joey would always wake her up. She started reading a book about animals and the afterlife given by a friend, and although very skeptical at first, it suddenly hit her deep in her soul that Joey was going to come back to find her.

When she contacted me for help to communicate with Joey's soul, I profoundly felt that he was going to come back in a similar body (because he really loved his body) of a Persian kitten but cream color with orange highlights instead of grey, and reunite with mom in about three months. I encouraged mom to let go of control, to continue to live fully each day while waiting for him, to trust the Universe and to let the magic manifest all in good time. It was a very difficult process and mom kept hoping he would just make it easy and show up at her front door.

Exactly three months later, I woke up with mom on my mind, which always means I'm about to hear from this person. Indeed, mom contacted me to tell me that she had an urge to look for a six-week old kitten online, but instead found an eleven-week old male cream Persian with orange highlights. The breeder lived about an hour away but was coming to town that day and could deliver him to her front door within a few hours. The speed at which Joey, now Fritz, came back was unbelievably amazing! Before mom or I could spend too much time thinking and analyzing the situation, the Universe and its powerful flow of energy had reunited two inseparable souls. As soon as mom opened the carrier door, Fritz purred and hugged her, then walked around the house like he already knew where everything was. His behavior has been very similar to Joey's in many ways, as he sleeps in the same spots at the same times of the day, and has the same playful personality. One night as he was playing, he jumped off the couch and while running over to a chair, mom saw fur that fell out of him, although it was a distinct clump of Joey's fur, which mom had not seen since he had passed. We believe it was Joey saying: "I'm back, Mom!"

Those are memorable and comforting experiences that help heal the heartache caused by losing such dear friends. Indeed, everyone takes a piece of our heart with them when they leave us and the pain can be extremely difficult to bear. To help heal and find peace, I ask each of my loved ones to fill my heart with love from the spirit world, and I remind myself of how blessed I am for having shared so many precious moments with so many magnificent souls, so that my heart doesn't feel broken but instead overflows with infinite love.

Chapter 6

A Whirlwind of Synchronicity, Warnings and Messages

In order to help as many people as possible assess their own life and areas of imbalances, prevent accidents, and keep or regain their health, I am listing a series of events that I attracted over the years, filled with wisdom from the animals. Fortunately, my awareness allowed me to recognize and understand them quickly, so I was able to make the right decisions, shift the energy, and keep myself on the right path of evolution to become wiser and more balanced. I recommend that we all pay attention because nature and animals often have a very unique message for us at a very specific time.

1. Balance always

While I was deciding that it was a smart decision to leave my phone on through the night, twenty-four hours a day, to help a colleague with being on call, Fuzz ran playfully at full speed towards me and freakishly misjudged his stopping distance, therefore plowing into me and flipping me on my back. I fell so hard that it is a miracle I did not break something. Mistake: wrong thinking and lack of boundaries pushed me out of balance. Key to salvage it: I declined helping my colleague and shut off my phone. My bruised back healed rapidly.

2. Stay on your true path

I almost stepped on a rattlesnake while walking randomly in the yard as I was wrongly thinking, again, that I should help a friend, even though it meant dishonoring some of my core values and principles. Thank you, Mr. Rattlesnake, for scaring me back onto the right path and helping me focus on what matters the most in life, which is respecting my boundaries and values as well as honoring myself. I must not disappoint myself and forget who I am. I must be true to myself first by learning to say no to others.

Many women (but also men) I have met are, like me, Mothers of the Earth. One doesn't need human children to be a great mother or to nurture. Mothers of the Earth take care of their neighbors, stray animals or people needing help. We basically try to take care of the whole planet and we find it hard (and sometimes impossible) to say no. Mothers of the Earth often feel responsible for others' emotions and want to fix it all for them. By doing this, they often lose dangerous amount of life energy and even lose themselves completely. It is hard to accept that we must let the world crumble and let everyone stumble and learn at their own pace. We want to save everyone else so badly, but our job is only to save ourselves and to respect others' ability to find their own way. You can't prevent someone from going through pain and you can't live someone else's life for them (and you couldn't do it as well as them anyway because you are not them and you don't have their gifts). You can only live your life and make your decisions to achieve balance, and have no regret in how much you give to others and how much you keep for yourself. However, you can hold someone else's hand while he or she goes through pain, and you can have your hand held while you go through pain.

In order to save ourselves, we must learn to love ourselves. Self-love means setting boundaries and only accepting who and what makes us happy in our life. We need to teach others how to treat us, what we will and will not accept. This is very difficult for caring and selfless people to do. We need to learn to care as much about ourselves as we care about others. This process includes grieving. We must grieve others and the whole world by making peace with what is and letting go of everything we wish was, and everything we want to change but cannot change. This is very freeing. I accept that I am only one grain of sand in a world of billions of grains of sand, and I am proud of my humble, yet so important, part and all the good I am doing. I decrease my interest in what I think others should be doing and I lower my expectations towards them. I want to die with a smile and be satisfied with what I have done. I choose to live with a smile because the more I do, the better and happier the world is.

We learn a lot from wild animals. They bring us back to the essence of life. They help us get back on track. A wild mother's priority is to save herself and the babies she can save, which means sometimes she must abandon a baby that is too weak to keep up the pace. It is sad but it is the law of the jungle for survival, otherwise everyone dies. Sometimes, humans must also make what is the hardest decision in life for caring people, which is to let a loved one fend for himself in order to save yourself. Choose life and keep moving forward, or stay behind and die.

3. Be You

I was walking around the yard in Arizona feeling defeated for not being able to just be myself around some colleagues. I felt shameful for being different and wished to be like everyone else, to blend in and make no waves. An impressive Saguaro cactus reminded me at that very moment to value myself and to take care of myself no matter when. I walked under one of its large arms and came up at the perfect time to push about a dozen large needles into my back. Two of them mistakenly stayed in for two weeks until they finally migrated out without complications thankfully. People who are different leave impressions on others. I had plenty of time to realize how good it felt to be me and appreciate my uniqueness. Each animal has a very unique nature as well. The bat, for example, is the only mammal that flies. In addition, every single bat has a very special personality. We all must honor our unique nature.

4. Protect yourself

I met with three people who were offering me a business opportunity, which I was unsure about accepting. When I got home that night, I found a scorpion, a black widow and a poisonous toad waiting for me at the door, representing the three people. Needless to say, I declined the offer.

A few years later, after being well behaved for many months, our pig Wilbur began finding ways to escape our property. He made us re-fence our few acres of land. This activity turned out to be very therapeutic as it reinforced our inner walls of protection as well. When I see a change in one of my animals' behavior, I always figure out what the message is, how we have become out of balance and how to readjust ourselves.

5. Follow the energy flow

I was invited by two wonderful old classmates to join them in Las Vegas and although I was very busy, I missed them dearly and wanted to see them. I hadn't seen them in over ten years. I had just helped a sweet lady say good bye to her two furry best friends at home. Before I left, she gave me a gorgeous and fancy shirt to thank me for my loving help. Receiving this shirt was the most appropriate synchronicity to tell me to go to Las Vegas, wear this beautiful shirt and have fun! Excited, I called my friends who asked me to make reservations for a show and dinner. After I booked what seemed to be the best show as well as the best vegan restaurant, I realized that both venues were in the same hotel, next to each other, which made it very easy. All was meant to be and the energy was flowing. We had a wonderful time!

6. Coexist in peace and harmony

I was hanging out in the yard at sunset and found eight black widows on their webs all around the house. Night time is when they come out to eat. Needless to say, I was destabilized and frightened, and knew that everybody I would talk to about it would tell me to kill them. However, I chose instead to make a pact with all eight black widows. I walked up to every single one repeating: "Leave me alone, I'll leave you alone, we can coexist in peace and harmony". They would hide during the day and come out at night. I minded my own business and they never hurt me in the eleven years we shared the beautiful desert of Arizona. We respected and tolerated one another. We should all learn to share the territory instead of wasting energy fighting.

7. Value your own life

I have been saving dragonflies that mistakenly visit the screened porch and are unable to find their way back out. I built a routine where I approach them calmly and gently pick them off the screen and into my hands to escort them out to freedom. To thank me, they now visit me and will land on my hands frequently when I am in the yard. One stared at me for many minutes while resting on my hand. I observed her in amazement while making memorable videos and taking pictures.

I told her how much I valued her life and how grateful I was for her presence on Earth. Then I heard her repeating to me: "I value your life, your life is precious and matters a great deal". I was touched by her reminding me that my life is unique, that there was never anyone else like me before and that there will never be anyone else like me after I die. Wow, it is truly my duty to share my gifts with the world. I owe it to myself. It is truly my reason for existing.

8. Show the world your beautiful colors

Following the guidance of the dragonflies, I started taking concrete actions to push myself out of my comfort zone, daring to shine my brightest. It did not take long to run into another powerful messenger, a magnificent Luna moth, who came out of the darkness of the night to show me his beautiful colors and tell me: "Yes! The time has arrived for you to also get out of the darkness and show the world how beautiful you are".

I realized that no matter what the outside world looks like, good or terrible, my power and purpose remain the same. I must dare showing my colors and share my gifts with the world, knowing that I can't control how they are received. I am not in control of their impact, great or small, which I can't fully measure. My job is to shine and let go of the rest. Focus on being the best you can be, even if the world seems hopeless. Don't let that paralyze you. Don't ever give up hope. Everyday, give your best effort and show the world how beautiful you are. By doing so, you are transforming the world and making it more beautiful.

9. Sometimes, the best decision is to do nothing

Many years ago, my husband and I went through a period of wanting to make a drastic life change, which included moving. It is easy to wonder if life would be better elsewhere. Obviously, the grass is not always greener on the other side, but sometimes it is, hence the confusion. Thankfully, a visitor came to our rescue and advised that we should stay in place for a while longer. That visitor was a large desert tortoise, the only one we got to see during our many years in

Arizona. It visited our two cats and me for almost an hour. I was mesmerized by the calmness of this tortoise progressing slowly but surely through life. She was the pure incarnation of not making any harsh move or drastic decision. She guided us to take it slowly, to make only small changes over time, and to believe that we would reach our destination. We followed this amazing creature's guidance.

10. What you do today will impact the world for millions of years to come

Walking our beautiful Florida land with our animals is the best therapy I know. Nature and wildlife are always present, selflessly sharing messages of guidance to those listening. The numerous tall and gorgeous trees make us feel hidden in an enchanted forest. The lush and green grass hides the most amazing treasures of seashells, reminding us how our whole property was submerged under the sea many millions of years ago. Our large spring-fed pond is the home of many fish, fresh water snails and turtles.

One day, I was standing in our sandy driveway and happened to stare at the broken shells when I found another amazing treasure: a large shark tooth that belonged to a megalodon. Megalodons lived over 3.5 million years ago and were the largest sharks. All of a sudden, my life became connected to the life of this giant of the sea, as we both shared the same home, only at different times on Earth.

Wow, I was speechless. I felt myself traveling through the cosmos at the speed of light, witnessing the evolution of planet Earth through its billions of years of life. What I do today, how I choose to live my life, will impact the life of other beings for millions and billions of years to come. We have a huge responsibility to protect our world and leave it in a better state than we found it.

11. The circle of life, we are ONE, WE are the web of life

Ever since I was a little girl, my dream has always been to travel the world as a missionary to bring peace on Earth. As I became older, I had to grieve the fact that my dream was too dangerous to accomplish but that I could still help a lot by remaining safe in the United States and Canada.

Many dangerous events that occurred at the Mexico-Arizona border over the years reminded me of it. Additionally, after making strong connections in Africa, the country became more violent than ever. I had to make peace with the sad fact that I wouldn't get to work closely with lions, tigers and elephants… well, until they all found me in Florida.

To my own amazement, I became the center of the circle, the circle of life, where I am home, where all life forms help one another, where all the animals from the kingdom unite and surround me with love and gratitude for my care and compassion towards all living beings. The strong energetic connections and karmic attractions that form in the web of life from our actions and intentions are unbelievably real and do come back to us, for better or worse.

When we moved into our home, we had no idea that we lived very close to a refuge for wild exotic animals. In fact we are so close that we not only hear them from our yard, but I now am privileged to help lions, tigers, jaguars, wolves, bears, lynx, African porcupine, deer and many more creatures live better by dispensing medications and performing lifesaving surgeries, as well as help them die better with humane euthanasia.

This manifestation of the circle of life in my life convinces me to remain awake, aware and mindful to create only positive energetic and karmic shifts around me. We reap what we sow.

12. Perseverance + Seizing opportunities = Luck

Living life with this attitude brings abundance and prosperity indeed. Going where the flow of energy is going and not forcing anything that offers great resistance (and therefore may not be beneficial), is another recipe to follow for happiness. When the time came to buy a camper to keep us mobile and safe during hurricane season, the right one literally fell in our lap. It also came with the most appropriate messenger of good fortune, a tiny ladybug that traveled on it all the way home seeming to say: "Good job, well done, you deserve this, enjoy!"

Connecting the dots can be very tricky until we have gone through many of them (life experiences) and now can see how much they all tie in together. That is why it is important to trust the unknown, persevere, seize opportunities and go with the flow that will connect the dots for us, even when we don't necessarily understand yet where we are going. It will become clearer later and we will be rewarded for our efforts.

13. We are stronger together

I have witnessed first-hand how predators like coyotes hunt as a team. One of them will venture away and tease a dog while the rest of the pack hides until it follows him back where it will be killed and eaten by the pack. Prey animals like wild horses or deer are also stronger together. When a predator approaches, the first one that sees him will shout the alarm sound and everyone will run away together to escape, often hiding the weak and the young in the middle of the pack to survive.

Humans need to learn that fighting among ourselves is detrimental to our survival. We have to work as a team. Migratory birds fly together. The bird in the front position has the toughest and most exhausting job as it must brave the wind. Birds rotate positions so everyone can relax at the back of the flock. In addition to teamwork, migratory birds also teach us to get out of the house, see the world, get out of our comfort zone, go for adventures, experience the world and learn from new environments.

14. Take time to play

All animals take time to have fun. It fuels the body and mind with good energy and reduces stress. Laugh with yourself when you embarrass yourself. Don't take yourself too seriously. Play with your pets and your loved ones, spend time with them. Time means love to our pets and our loved ones. Money can't buy back the time we wasted doing a million other things and not sharing quality time with the ones we love the most. Remember to laugh and be silly with them while you still can. Playing keeps us young at heart and rejuvenates our whole being.

15. Be a gentle giant

Like the tigers, use your strength and life energy wisely, only for what matters, which is to survive. Just because you can kill a human, an animal, an insect or a plant, it doesn't mean that you should. Tigers in captivity enjoy spending their energy going for walks with their human caretakers. They also choose to swim and jump up and down, even the old ones, thanks to some amazing pain relievers. They also spend it roaring in unison during the passing of a fellow tiger, giving their support and escorting their old companion into the next world. Don't waste your life energy having a negative impact on the world. Save it to do good around you. Be a gentle giant.

16. Remain aware of your surroundings at all times

Wolves teach us to not trust anyone. No one is perfect. Many people will disappoint or fail you even when they don't mean to. Trust your instincts and stay on your guards. When you give your power to someone else and you know you shouldn't have, you only have yourself to blame.

17. Invest in the next generation

Most animals must invest time and energy in teaching their young how to survive, hunt, fly and be! Most humans are too busy making money to invest themselves fully in teaching and training the young in their care. Most humans want the magic pill that will teach and raise their pets and children miraculously, without having to spend time doing it. Consequently, we are sadly seeing the degeneration of the future generations: young animals and people lacking the needed guidance to make better choices, getting neglected, lost and wounded emotionally and physically, in turn neglecting and harming others, including the next generation they are supposed to guide but are unable to.

Elephants share a huge amount of maternal love, wisdom and critical thinking through generations, which is the key for survival of the species. The human race would do well to follow their guidance.

18. We are a product of our environment

Our environment defines us. We are only as good as the environment we are in. If a plant doesn't grow and thrive, we need to improve its living conditions. The same applies for people and animals. The better our environment, the better we are. Many animals and people are dying because their environment is dying. Let's set them up for success.

19. Adaptability

Like the octopus and the chameleon, adapt to any situation, make the best of it and learn from it. Remain flexible physically, mentally and emotionally, which increases your resilience and performance through life.

20. Be resourceful

Follow the example of rabbits and do it yourself. Rabbits love to be in charge of their own life. They love to build their home and burrows as well as organize their surroundings and build a daily routine. Don't look for answers outside yourself about how to live. Find skills inside yourself and develop them so you don't depend on others. Develop your creativity and become resourceful. Think outside the box!

Chapter 7

Pitfalls of Domestication

Creators of sustainable immigration reform for humans could draw a lot of wisdom from feral cat colonies. The bottom line is that as much as anyone might want to save all the cats of the world, there is not enough room to bring them all in one's home. The territory is limited, and overcrowding it beyond what is sustainable will lead to fights and chaos. The same concept applies to bringing an overwhelming number of immigrants to a new country. Once again, balance is the key. If everyone could limit themselves to bringing just a few cats into their homes, and if every country would bring a few immigrants into their territory, we would help greatly. What more can we do? Let's fix the root cause of the problem. Let's help feral cats thrive in their own environment and help people thrive in their own country. Let's provide birth control to stop breeding and stabilize the populations with the basic needs of water, food, shelter, sleep, safety and medical care. Then, let's empower everyone to take better care of themselves.

Along the same wavelengths, many conservationists want to transport large exotic animals, such as elephants, giraffes, lions and tigers, from their countries of origin to safer countries to save the species and prevent extinction. The idea is absolutely noble but unfortunately, the same rules apply. Humans can take over for Mother Nature and save a few lives, however, it only takes a few elephants who can live up to seventy-five years in captivity, each eating hundreds of pounds of food daily, to overwhelm the situation and make it completely unsustainable. Moreover, when it comes to reproduction, we need a large number of animals to ensure that we breed better genetics and healthier animals and not the opposite. We can't possibly measure up to Mother Nature. How can we fix the root cause of this problem? The answer remains the same: focus on providing a safe environment for these magnificent animals in their own habitat. Their habitat must be protected which will provide them with water, food, shelter, sleep and safety. We can then provide medical care and facilitate breeding to reverse the damage done by humans who have destroyed too many animals and their habitat. Let's bring back biodiversity and rewild the world.

The question is: can we be fast enough to stop the human race from destroying the planet? The answer will be revealed in the next few years, based on how humans decide to go forward. Our situation is extremely dire considering the other problem on our hands, the human and domesticated animal overpopulation crisis, which is aggravated by the total disregard of any attempt at breeding only the healthiest individuals in order to obtain the healthiest offspring, as discussed in my first book. This is especially concerning since most domesticated animals are dogs and cats eating carnivorous diets, on top of most humans consuming animal products, which has led to the destruction of most forests and lands turned into farms. Humans then kill billions of wild animals to protect the ones they farm and spend more time, money and resources feeding those animals than they would spend feeding a plant-based diet to the entire world population. We must stop farming animals and go vegan. We must stop destroying our environment and grow more trees. The most touching present that I have ever received was a tree that a very grateful pet owner planted in my honor, how precious! Let's spread the word!

What did humans and animals gain from domestication? Many things, which are worth discussing. The idea was great from the very beginning: developing a partnership between humans and wolves to facilitate hunting and get a reliable food source, share shelter, increase protection as well as providing companionship. It was a win-win situation. It made life easier for all. The bond continued to develop until it became what it is today. The advantages of domestication in our modern world remain: a reliable food source, protection, sharing shelter and companionship.

Companionship takes on a whole new meaning in our modern world as animals give people what people have lost the ability to give to one another. Animals are supporting us emotionally and filling the holes by giving us their unconditional love, time, patience, forgiveness and support. They believe in us even when we don't believe in ourselves and they make us feel valued. Animals never judge us allowing us to just be. They are truthful and real, they help us live simply and in the now, and they make us look at the bright side of life. They teach us gratitude, how to be happy and how to reconnect with nature, with the Source and with what matters in life. Animals teach us balance, to slow down and play, to smell the flowers and to take time to stretch. They make us get up in the morning and exercise, they teach us resilience and they keep us going. Domestication has allowed animals to experience life very differently than they would have in the wild and has given them different life missions and purposes.

Where did we go wrong? Domestication has also created new challenges as many animals have taken on our human problems and become out of balance: not spending enough time outside and a modern sedentary lifestyle have created an obesity crisis, constipation, boredom, feelings of disconnection from nature and of losing one's purpose as well. Many animals take on our emotional burden and our stress of living, which leads to diseases and behavioral issues that they would not have experienced in the wild.

Moving the body is so important yet so overlooked. Animals remember the need to move, which is crucial for a good digestion.

Unfortunately, humans often can't provide the amount of exercise needed for their animals' mind, body and soul to feel good. Furthermore, many animals are forced to spend many hours a day confined in cages and some even spend their whole lives in cages. This is the case for too many domesticated rabbits and it is unacceptable. Rabbits still have an amazingly strong instinct of survival, of finding their own food and of building their homes and burrows. They are extremely smart and inquisitive. They need room to move, hop around and enjoy life. There is nothing more gratifying than to watch them graze all day long like nature intended for them to do.

For people looking for motivation to move and exercise, my best advice is to go pick up a caged up shelter dog and exercise together in nature, instead of locking yourself in artificial conditions in a gym. Your life and your new companion's life will be changed forever and for the better.

As discussed earlier, in an ideal world we would find that perfect balance between the wild and domestic lifestyles that would provide safety, fulfillment and sustainability for all animals and humans. This concept brings us back to living more like Native Americans did, by respecting and protecting nature, living in harmony with the web of life, drastically reducing breeding of humans and domesticated animals, and facilitating breeding of wild animals to help re-balance their populations and avoid extinction.

Unfortunately, failure to do this has already created an alarmingly excessive number of cats, who are fierce hunters and who have caused the decimation of many wild bird populations. Bird lovers tell cat lovers to keep those predators inside, which we know is not always in the cats' best interest. Humans have also contributed to the death of many birds by their use of pesticides, their pollution with plastic, their need for buildings with big windows that birds collide with, their monoculture farming practices and their removal of native plants to grow lawns that don't offer enough food or shelter for many birds. Nature is far better than humans at controlling populations via its predator-prey population cycles.

We should eat healthy and sustainably vegan, which means gardening or else picking our organic fruits and veggies from sustainable farms practicing regenerative agriculture, and not from giant farms that destroy everything to grow their foods as it is the case with palm oil. Orangutans are suffering greatly from palm oil harvest, which is used in countless numbers of food products that we really don't even need. There are plenty of alternatives to palm oil and ways to harvest it sustainably if need be. The same goes for chocolate and coffee companies that are also very destructive. Let's read the labels and read about the food companies that we choose to support. Look for the Rainforest Alliance Certified logo as well as the Fair Trade Certified logo that support fair treatment of workers and no work slavery among children. Let's extend our efforts to buying products from local sources as much as possible to reduce carbon footprint and waste due to transportation. We should also be able to follow the companies' practices closely for transparency and integrity.

Luckily, as discussed before, vegan diets for cats and dogs are also now appearing on the market, which will greatly help with sustainability. Culturing meat in a lab might also be a reality some day. If one really feels the need to eat animal meat, insects are by far the healthiest, lowest cruelty practice, and the most economical and environmentally friendly way to go! Enjoy, and be on the look out for insect-based diets appearing on the market for dogs and cats as well!

If we stopped breeding domestic animals today, in less than twelve years we would have fixed the pet overpopulation problem since most domesticated animals live an average of ten to fifteen years. Let's do our best so that when we die, we will be able to tell ourselves that we gave it our all.

Chapter 8

More about your essence

We hurt the way we are, which means that our body follows our mind and our personality in how it gets sick or hurt. Many holistic dentists, such as Dr. Genevieve Desloges in the book *Les dents nous parlent (Teeth speak to us)*, describe the different relationships between our teeth and our emotions, organs, meridians and personality traits. See if any of this relates to you and your situation. Look at your front top two teeth:

1. The Judge/The Sheriff—has SHARP TRIANGULAR shaped teeth. He has many opinions on everything and an inflexible mind. He tries to fix everything and calls others out on things they are not doing perfectly. He is intolerant, he implements rules and dresses in black and white. He often has fast acute diseases such as fracturing a tooth or bone. He is prone to joint stiffness and circulatory blockages.

2. The Athlete—has SHARP SQUARED shaped teeth. He has a powerful physique and an over-the-top reactive mind and body. He is often very competitive, impatient, stressed, angry, aggressive and impulsive. He is afraid of being the weakest, losing or being dominated, and he often revolts. He believes he must always win and be the strongest. He gets acute over-the-top diseases such as raging tooth infection, high fever and allergies to medications or sutures.

3. The Pleaser—has SMOOTH SQUARED shaped teeth.

He has a pretty smile and teeth and doesn't dare expressing his feelings. He holds everything in, boils inside and builds thick walls to hide his true self. He often develops thick-walled cysts as well as slow and chronic gum and body inflammation.

4. The Lover—has ROUND shaped teeth. He has a bubbly personality and is compassionate. He needs others' attention, is very emotional and dependant. He is prone to cavities since he perceives his life as having holes from not enough love. He has hypersensitive gums and a low pain threshold.

5. The Artist—has SMOOTH TRIANGULAR shaped teeth. He loves colorful clothes, is anxious and tries to escape living in this crazy world by building a sweeter imaginary world. He is prone to gum recession because his gums are disappearing, going away, escaping just like his mind.

None of the above is set in stone and, just like dreams, diseases will have different meanings for different people. However, it is fascinating to link our teeth development (and the rest of our body) to our mind and personality. It even seems that our birth is influenced by our personality: a very determined person will have been born fast in one push or prematurely, someone who respects deadlines and is always on time will have been born right on schedule, someone who is fearful and hesitant to make decisions will have had a slow or delayed birth, or might have been forced out via cesarean section. I had a smooth, simple and happy birth according to my mother, which seems to represent adequately how I navigate through life. A fun fact about me is that I was born with a tooth already present in my mouth. We are still debating the meaning of this!

The goal is to achieve balance in our personality. For example, not only the Lover can develop cavities. Someone who feels oppressed, is unable to express himself freely and wants to bite back may develop multiple cavities. Someone who feels others are invading his personal space and is unable to build strong walls of protection may also develop multiple cavities. Again, it is about our personality and how our mind chooses to feel and react to life situations. Some people and animals are very dramatic and their medical history shows it, often including multiple emergency visits, acute illnesses, crises and freak accidents. The medical team must remain on the look out for them since things always seem to get out of control. Death for them is also usually dramatic unfortunately, since we often die the way we live.

People who are quick at making decisions, who know what they want, who move quickly through life, speak fast and are always on the go will typically have a quick death as well. On the other hand, those who speak slowly, walk slowly, do not make waves, take time to make any decisions and hesitate a lot in life will have plenty of time to prepare for their death. Their illnesses tend to develop slowly as well. If you describe your disease with words or explain how it makes you feel, you might find out what situation in your life caused it. The words you use might help you find the emotional root cause of it. For example, a friend who was feeling torn between two love relationships for years developed chronic skin tearing of her genital organs, and when she found closure emotionally and stopped feeling torn, her torn skin finally healed. I had a phase during which I felt very deflated and out of steam, meanwhile I kept getting flat tires on my car. The more we can figure out why diseases and trouble happen to us and to our animals, the better it is for our health and growth.

List all traumas, accidents, allergies, fears, illnesses, problems and challenges you and your pets have or had. Refer to my first book to figure out where you or your pet became out of balance: is it related to your diet? Lifestyle? Environment? Feeding off someone else? Getting your energy drained by someone? Related to a past life? Genetic? From stress or negative emotions? Not being in tune with your life mission? Part of your soul contract? What is your body telling you? Why did you attract it? Is it a blessing in disguise? Were you doing something for the wrong reasons? Wrong thinking? Wrong place? Famous last word? Were you judging? Did you jinx yourself? What is the message, the life lesson, the teaching to grow? Answer those questions with your brain, your heart and your gut, wherever the answer comes from.

A horse that hates competing might get hurt all the time. Someone who hates their job might also get sick enough to not be able to work, like a tired massage therapist I know who accidentally sliced her thumb and finally got the time off she needed to rest. Pets often get sick because they swim in their owners' low vibrating energy and toxic emotions. Our words are powerful. I avoid saying things like: "You are a pain in my butt". Jinxes are also truly powerful. I avoid snap judgments of others because they can come back to test us and see how much better we do in someone else's situation. If you feel a bad vibe, find out where it's coming from and shift the energies right away to make it disappear by taking action or changing your thought process.

Both my shadow Fuzz and I have allergies, eye issues and are vegan. We are both goofy, love to have fun and are also very astute. We have a ton of freckles, share the same light brown hair color and were meant to share life together. My husband and his canine shadow Yogi share a whole other set of characteristics. They are very emotional beings, they prefer the comfort of home to any social situation and both need meat in their diets. Their connection is such that they also look similar with their black hair. Here are a few pointers that may apply to some people and animals.

Brain cancer: for over-thinkers and over-achievers who always have too much on their plate, they are growing more brain cells to help them solve all their problems and get all their work done. It is imperative to mention the overuse of cell phones that emit toxic electromagnetic radiation causing brain cancer as well.

Breast cancer: maternal conflict or fear of not being a good mother. A cat losing her kittens may develop breast cancer trying to produce more milk while mourning and looking for her kittens. A woman who can't become pregnant or who has a conflicting relationship with a child can also develop breast cancer.

Allergies/sneezing: when you can't stand your situation or environment and are rejecting it.

Genital organs issues: lack of self-esteem and self-image, loss of masculine or feminine power, feeling ashamed of not being a good enough man or woman. A person who suffers from incest or rape may perceive her/his genital organs as dirty and sex as bad, and develop cancer.

Constipation: holding in something, resisting something, not wanting to let go. For some animals and people, like our cat Sunny and human friend Kathi, not having the freedom to spend more time outside, feeling blocked, will lead to this physical manifestation.

Vomiting/Diarrhea: rejecting a situation, like the many dogs being boarded away from home who don't want to be there, as opposed to those who enjoy themselves and remain healthy. As discussed in my first book, our cat Munchie violently rejected the situation of another cat moving in and developed vomiting and diarrhea.

Bladder trouble: territorial issues. A cat not allowed outside might get upset that he is restricted to a small territory and get a bladder blockage. A lady I know developed a urinary tract infection during her divorce when she had to move out and lost her territory. Someone else experienced the same illness when she lost her job, therefore her place.

Heart disease: feeling heart-broken from any situation

causing intense sadness and powerlessness, such as being separated from a loved one. Also when someone feels rejected from a situation that he cherished deeply or got pushed away from being in charge of a project.

Stomach issues: when one can't digest bad news or is overwhelmed by too much to process.

Mouth and throat issues: when one is unable to express himself and communicate adequately.

Weight issues: some people and animals may be overweight because, on a subconscious level, they don't feel seen or else they are trying to protect themselves or a loved one, therefore they gain weight to be seen and be more intimidating. Skinny people and animals may try to disappear because they feel unwanted or have no place.

Eye issues: changing reality to make it more bearable to watch.

Ear issues: when one doesn't want to hear any toxic sounds like loved ones fighting. Married to a man who couldn't communicate calmly, Sarah's body started producing excessive ear wax to the point of causing partial deafness to block her spouse's annoying and loud arguments. She confronted him and taught him to control his emotions and lower his voice, which healed her ears over a few years. My friend Sheila chose to be born deaf after experiencing the awful sounds of war in her previous life.

Lung issues: feeling choked by someone or a situation, in current life or from a past life.

The goal in figuring out why diseases or obstacles occur in our life is obviously to help us and our animals feel better and be healthier, to grow and improve our outlook and attitude towards life, and to be at our best to shine our brightest. However, let's remember that even healthy animals and people die because we all do. The body will fail us at some point and death will happen, most commonly on our birthday as research has shown, which makes a lot of sense. Leaving the Earth the same day we arrived and coming full circle. Therefore, we should regularly turn off our brain, stop analyzing and focus on just enjoying the wonderful ride of being alive while it lasts. We need to be patient and make peace with any illness or unpleasant situation happening because we are learning from it. We need to stabilize the sick body by sending it love, combined with any helpful healing modality. We must believe that the situation is temporary and separate ourselves from it, as a disease is not our identity and it doesn't define who we are. We need to focus on healing and we need to thank the disease or situation for helping us grow.

I find it important to discuss the power of our hair. Science has proven that the hair covering our head and body is an extension of our nervous system. I see each of them as an antenna feeling the world around us. Furthermore, science has proven that people with long hair tend to be less tired, more energetic and less likely to become depressed. The bones in the forehead are porous and function to transmit light to the pineal gland, which affects brain activity as well as thyroid and sexual hormones. Cutting bangs, which cover the forehead, impedes this process and also inhibits intuition by covering our third eye chakra. Military personnel have noticed the power of long hair (as well as the loss of power of short hair) and confirmed what many indigenous cultures have known for a long time: the longer your antennas, the more inner power and intuition you have to feel your way through life. Native Americans further believe that long hair connects us to nature, life consciousness and spirit, in addition to having extrasensory perceptions, which I fully agree with. To our biggest surprise, both my husband's and my long hair even curls like powerful energy vortexes.

Chapter 9

Clean up your life often

At the end of each calendar year, I routinely lighten the load in all aspects of my life. I finish as many projects as possible and fix everything I can that is not feeling right so that I can start the New Year as clear and as Zen as possible. I also make it a point to clean up each life chapter ending in order to get maximum closure and leave the past behind.

In addition, each day deserves a dose of cleaning and I accomplish that by spending time in nature with the sun, the trees and the grass, as well as by taking care of any uneasy feelings about anything right away. Listening to music, playing music, taking a shower, imagining a shower of white light cleansing any non-beneficial energies from my being and from my animals, swimming, putting my bare feet in the water, cutting energetic ties with toxic people or situations with an imaginary knife, smudging with white sage and pine as well as holding a selenite crystal are all great ways to cleanse and lighten the load.

Luckily, many shamans and energy workers are available to help us with major cleanings as well. When I feel the need for extra protection, I imagine wrapping myself in a bubble of white light, I cross my legs and arms and I call upon fierce animal spirits to keep me safe. Starting fresh at any point in life is also extremely empowering. Reinventing yourself requires courage as it brings challenges and fears to overcome, but the results of freedom, power and happiness are well worth the efforts. As I said before, ending the Arizona life chapter was the hardest thing I have ever done. I had no other options since I had become such a prisoner, and without a doubt, the freedom I gained from this difficult challenge saved my life.

Just like a lobster, I had outgrown my shell, which had become tight and uncomfortable. Although changes are scary, resisting them can be extremely dangerous. In order to continue growing, I had to become vulnerable, shed my shell, leave it behind and dare transform into the new me for this next life chapter.

I learned when I was very young to “play the game of life”. It helps me see difficulties in life very differently from most people. I have learned to welcome them and embrace them because they are often my biggest blessings and opportunities for growth. Daring to jump off the cliff and become destabilized leads to amazing new experiences. Indeed, my imaginary wings have always appeared. I have the most supportive husband, parents, parents-in-law, and my animals have always saved me as well! Animals have inspired me to be resilient like they are, to never give up, to keep moving forward, to have gratitude and to always believe in a brighter tomorrow.

Hence, it is very exciting when I clean up and remove anything or anyone from my life who is no longer helpful to my evolution or who has become toxic. Blood relatives, famous or important people with important job functions in society, everyone is on the same level when it comes to protecting yourself. If there is anyone in my life with baggage, drama or issues that are not mine to fix or to deal with, I give it all back to them, I remove them from my life and I close the door on the past.

Unfortunately, a soul’s karmic debt or else family karma still must be dealt with as a part of one’s life mission. Both often appear as a theme or repetitive obstacle in one’s life, or are present in many succeeding generations that different family members must face until finally someone transcends it. I have learned to, once again, embrace the valuable lessons and good that are attached, which helps me to get through the painful process. This can look like a separation between a parent and children, adultery, addiction or domestic violence. Again, it helps to put these situations into perspective from a non-emotional observer standpoint and understand that we could not have avoided them because they are a part of something much bigger than ourselves that we can't control. Overcoming a karmic debt or family karma is a powerful accomplishment as it changes you and your lineage for generations to come.

Some behaviors and ways of thinking we might have had for many years can also finally catch up with us when we reach a point of knowing better and we become forced to improve our ways and behaviors. The life lesson comes to the forefront of our life and we can no longer escape it without something going wrong. For example, someone who used to make a living as a lumberjack gets hurt and can no longer cut trees. After the initial shock, he embraces his new and improved next life chapter by planting trees for living and saving the Earth, as well as teaching others to do the same. We shared a similar experience with our cat Munchie many years ago. She had been eating the same diet for years until she developed chronic vomiting. It prompted us to not only start reading cat food labels more attentively but all human food labels as well. That was the ultimate turning point when we made a big life change and drastically improved all of our diets by removing many preservatives, chemicals, pesticides, by-products, additives like salt and sugar, suboptimal and processed foods. We are what we eat. Raw, fresh, organic, low glycemic foods, sprouted whole grains, nuts, seeds and legumes are best. A cleaner body vibrates at a higher energetic frequency and has a stronger life force. A cleaner body rejuvenates and means healthier intestines, better digestion, a healthier mind and more brainpower as well.

What does your diet say about you? List the ten food items

that you eat the most. Can you do better? Is it time to clean up your plate and feed your body better foods? What cravings do you have and what emotions are they triggered by (caffeine, sweet, salty, starchy, fatty foods)? We all eat our emotions at times so it is very helpful to pay attention to them in order to fix them, not with food because it never truly fills the void, but with true food for the soul such as love, support, respect, fulfillment, happiness, confidence, feeling heard and valued. For more on this topic, you may enjoy reading Doreen Virtue's book titled *Constant Craving*. Meanwhile, healing cravings is a process so be patient with yourself. A good starting point for most people is to focus on eating less by putting smaller portions in our plate and using a smaller plate so it looks full. Taking time to chew our food and eating slowly also helps greatly. Listen to your stomach and stop eating when it tells you it is full. When you feel extremely hungry or you have a craving, start with a fruit or vegetable and drink water. It is amazing how quickly we feel full when we listen to our stomach.

Another rule I live by is not to waste any food. Even the smallest leftover food is tasty later on or the next day. When I go to a restaurant, I make sure to decline all straw, plastic utensils, plastic bags and I even bring my own reusable containers. Some waiters may look at me like I come from another planet but that's ok, I know Mother Nature thanks me and I hope to set an example for others to follow. I also make a leftover plate for Wilbur with items such as potato peels and other foods that would end up thrown away. Living a zero-waste lifestyle teaches us gratitude for what we have.

Let's reflect upon the closest people and animals supporting you and supporting one another.

- Who is in your Family Unit? List the most significant animals or humans, on Earth or in Heaven, with whom you navigate through life and death.

- Are the beings around me right? Are my current Family Unit members all beneficial for me and for one another in this current life chapter?
- Are the people and animals that we interact with, outside our Family Unit, beneficial for us?
- Who makes you feel polluted/angry/upset/drained/exhausted/jinxed? What toxic relationships exist around you?
- Who makes you feel loved, safe and comforted?
- Who makes you feel both good and bad?

It is important to make sure that all our relationships are beneficial, which doesn't necessarily mean they are easy. As discussed before, animals and people on our path will help us grow, which can be an extremely difficult process. Our pets can also have difficult but beneficial relationships among themselves, as they share growth opportunities and important life lessons for their evolution. The sooner we embrace the process, we stop resisting it and we try our best to overcome the challenges (knowing that we will keep attracting them until we do), the better it is for all involved and the rewards will be greater than we could have ever imagined.

Relationships are of different types and purposes among animals and humans. We attract them to help us grow and achieve balance. When it comes to human love relationships, I have witnessed people having a twin soul in their life multiple times. I define a twin soul as someone who resembles us immensely (even often physically!) and, consequently, with whom growth is limited. It is like being in a relationship with yourself, which makes you feel safe, at home and is very comforting. Twin souls make great and stable parents. Other twin souls seem to have made a pact to incarnate together young but then are kept at a healthy distance by invisible forces for most of their lives in order to have rich life experiences focused on personal growth by being in relationships with other people. Some twin souls reunite later in life but some don't. My good neighbor Mary lost hers when she was only three years old and still remembers today the pain she felt when he died. Even at such a young age, she understood what was going on as she cried disproportionately. My good friend Debbie lost her twin soul from suicide while they were both married to other people. Sadly, after she divorced, she moved back to her hometown where he was living but he had suffered too much to wait for her. She misses him greatly. Norma found the courage to leave her twin soul after a long relationship that became toxic, stunting them both in their evolution. Time will tell if they reunite later in life. Merry and her twin soul, Mike, did find each other in their sixties and it was love at first sight. They quickly became like two peas in a pod, totally and beautifully inseparable.

A different type of love relationship among humans is with a soulmate. This relationship is often challenging yet is the most rewarding. Soulmates have known each other since the spirit world. They complete each other and therefore are stronger together. They are meant to be in a relationship for the long haul even though, unfortunately, many don't stand the test of time. Their strength of being different is also their biggest challenge and often causes many sparks and arguments. They will push each other to their evolutionary limit, with maximum growth at maximum speed, which can be exhausting. No matter how many fights they have, invisible forces seem to always bring them back together. Their meaningful relationship requires a lot of effort in order to avoid judging, hurting and trying to change one another. Both need to remain focused on overcoming the tough life lessons they face while respecting and honoring each other's nature and differences, as well as focused on mastering the four most difficult skills of all: compassion, forgiveness, universal patience and unconditional love towards yourself and towards your partner. Those are essential to experience the most blissful accomplishment of self-realization. Soulmates who give up will jump from one unfulfilling relationship to another until they finally realize that they belong together, like my friend Susannah and her ex-husband (who is now her new boyfriend) did. Life is better together.

No matter what relationship we are in, let's try our best to respect and understand where our partner is coming from, which is often difficult since we all have a very unique past, therefore a unique perception of life according to our good and bad experiences that have created our beliefs, either limiting or empowering. Consequently, we all wear a unique pair of glasses. Let's try our best to understand and support one another with compassion, communicate openly without judgment, negotiate, fairly compromise and acknowledge each others' wounds to help them heal. Growing takes time. Each small step in the right direction should be celebrated. Let's teach one another the lessons we learned from past experiences and obstacles faced. Let's accept that no one is perfect and that mistakes will be made. Let's not dwell on them. Let's look ahead and keep moving forward. As long as both try hard to minimize them and fix them when they happen, let's forgive our partner and ourselves, and help one another grow and heal like two best friends, trying their best to be at their best. What more can one ask for? We must realize that our parents are also a product of their environment and life experiences. We must forgive them for their mistakes and make peace with the fact that they are not perfect either. Everyone was born clueless, everyone is here to grow, everyone will hurt themselves and others. The key is to never lose sight of the good in the one we love, to admire the good in him or her, and to continue to bring out the best in each other. Trust like you have never been let down and love like you have never been hurt. Every morning is a fresh start to reinvent yourself and your perception of the world with a better pair of glasses! Let's enjoy navigating on the ocean of life together.

What would make you, your pets, your spouse and your children feel more alive? You and your Family Unit vibrate to the level of what you focus on and what you surround yourself with. Make a list of everything that bugs you in your life and that you want to see disappear. Be honest with yourself in making the list. What do you want? Surround yourself with people that have good and uplifting energy. Remove people that are depleting your energy, damaging you, bringing you down and polluting you. Where do you or members of your Family Unit lose vital energy? Complaining? Comparing yourself to others? Being criticized for being different? Are your pets and children absorbing all your stress? Ask yourself to whom and to what am I choosing to give my vital energy to today? Be mindful of how you can do better. Write one change that you want in your life, one change that each of your pets wants, one change that your spouse wants, one change that each of your children wants, and take action now. If you think your pet hates his collar or hates his crate, let's make a change. I met Fiona, a little extremely fluffy Pomeranian who hated to be brushed. We successfully built a new routine by changing everything: the place, the time, the brush used, we even changed her owner's energies focusing on "spa day for the queen" as opposed to "torture session happening". We shifted the energies and Fiona followed along beautifully.

Do you live your life in fear or in love? Why do you do what you do? Dress up a certain way, make the bed a certain way, close all the blinds, for you or for others? Do you make your life decisions in fear (of others' rules or others' disapproval) or in love for yourself? Do your loved ones behave out of fear? Allow yourself to feel what you need to be you. Allow your loved ones to feel what they need to be themselves. Can you and everyone around you, people and animals, express themselves freely or are you suppressing one another? Do you take the time to speak with them? How can you improve your communication with everyone? How well do you know them? Do you think they are happy? What more can you do to make them happier or healthier? Pretend you are each of your loved ones and you are seeing the world through their eyes, what do you see? How does your loved one perceive you? How do you make each of them feel?

What else bugs you? Continue listing all the things in your life that bug you, that give you a knot in your stomach, that conflict you and stress you. Any regrets, guilt, things you wish you had done, done differently or not done, how can you fix them? Everyday make lists of feelings that are not right and fix them as you go. For example, write a letter to a departed loved one telling him what you wish you had told him before he died; write a letter to the soul of someone who is alive but who you don't feel comfortable confronting or speaking with; write a letter of love, compassion, forgiveness and encouragement to yourself as well as to your inner child; to heal emotional trauma from bad experiences, re-write the past the way you wish it happened, the way you wish bullies, siblings or parents acted, and the actions you wish you took. Re-write your life story. You can truly change the energies of the past and of your childhood to find closure and healing. Your mind can't tell the difference between what's real and what's not. Hug your inner child and hug yourself.

Write a list of what the world needs, of your passions and of your dreams and start making them come true. Lighten up mentally, emotionally, physically and materially. Your vital energy level will rise enormously and you will feel more alive and happy than ever!

Chapter 10

Light up the World

In the workshop that Bandito and I created, everyone is guided to reflect on his or her own life balance. We should ask ourselves these questions below often, as often as needed, even at the end of each day. What are my current needs and areas of imbalance? Using your brain and your heart, answer with either: no, not enough, too much, or yes I am in perfect balance and shining my brightest! Be honest with yourself, it is the first step in healing and growing.

- Am I comfortable with who I have become? Physically? Emotionally? Spiritually?
- How much am I being myself around others? Are all my needs being met?
- How much do I love myself? Is my inner child well cared for?
- How strong is my inner peace and protective bubble?
- Do I have enough fulfillment and purpose? Do I contribute enough to society?
- Do I take time to feed my soul with physical, mental and emotional stimulation?
- Do I have a routine?
- Do I get enough sleep?
- Do I have healthy social interactions?
- Do I have loving, caring and trusting relationships?

- Do I get enough physical love, hugs and kisses?
- Do I have support, stability and safety on all levels, emotional, physical and financial?
- Do I exercise, dance and move enough?
- Do I have fun? Do I play and laugh?
- Am I stressed, fearful or anxious?
- Do bullies, peer pressure and judgment from others affect me?
- Am I in pain?
- Was I at my place today? Am I at my place in this current life chapter?
- Do I feel alive (or am I dying, burning out, a life chapter is trying to close)?
- Is my work fulfilling? Is it me? Is it bringing out the best in me?
- Is my environment right for my current life chapter?
- Do my life, lifestyle, travels, friends and hobbies represent who I am? Is this me?

Look at yourself and your life from an outsider's perspective. Look at everything: your home, your living quarters, your furniture, your appliances, your decorations and your clothes. Are you happy when you look around? Do you enjoy your coffee table or does it remind you of your ex making you cringe inside every time you look at it? If so, give it away to someone who doesn't have any bad memories associated with it. That way you both get a fresh start; it's a win-win situation. Are your clothes and jewelry representative of who you are? If not, give them away. One man's trash is another man's treasure. Is your lifestyle representative of who you are? Doing the things we love and being who we are increases our vital energy level and life force.

If your pet likes to wear clothes, make sure they suit his or her personality. Color therapy is great! Give an orange harness or collar to a shy dog to help him socialize and come out of his shell, a blue bed to an anxious dog to bring him peace and calm (can be combined with lavender essential oil, music), and use red to bring vitality to an old companion. What color does your pet prefer?

I always laugh when I give directions to our home to close friends or family members. In order to get to our country home, one must drive through a very developed neighborhood where all the houses are the same, on minimal land with limited trees. Our guests are always relieved when they arrive, thinking they were lost because they couldn't believe we lived in such a developed area, until they finally saw our dirt road leading to our magical land filled with the most majestic trees representing us, then they knew it was right.

Indeed, some animals and people belong in the wild. Everyone must be comfortable living a life that is true to his or her identity. Everyone needs routine to some extent, even me! Most animals are happier with a routine as well. I have met quite a few frantic and exhausted dogs and cats trying to cope with their families' unpredictable schedules. One in particular, a ten-month-old Bichon named Petunia, was so stressed by the constant change in her owners' schedule that she would worry sick, become destructive and even vomit if they didn't come home before a certain time. The decision was made to re-home her with the owners' parents who lived a more stable life, which was the right decision. Her new lifestyle made her much more Zen with scheduled daily walks and mealtimes. She stopped vomiting and being destructive. I have met quite a few other animals for which the time came to change families because they no longer fit or thrived. One became the bully; another became bullied and buried under three more dominant dogs until his owner re-homed him at a friend's house where he became the only pet and was treated like a prince; another never really bonded with his owner who had saved his life and met a stranger with whom it was love at first sight. Whatever the reason may be, let's remain open to the signs of guidance and necessary changes from one life chapter to the next that will be beneficial for everyone involved.

Your environment should suit you and make you thrive. It needs to make your life energy flow. Are you and each of your pets living your best life? Repeatedly ask and answer all the above questions from the beginning of this chapter for all members of your Family Unit, animals and humans. For each pet ask yourself: does he or she belong indoor only, outside only, or some combination of both? Is boarding perceived as fun or stressful? Find everyone's new place to shine their brightest while they are here and make a lasting impact on our world even after they leave.

What are your hobbies? Do you thoroughly enjoy them? Or are you feeling peer pressure or the need to please or impress someone? What kind of TV shows do you watch, if any? Or do you leave your television play all day as background noise? Noise pollution, bombardment from advertisements and horror movies are tough on us and on our animals. I have met animals that suffered terrible stress and anxiety from them. Many people don't realize how much it affects them and their animals.

Are you spending too much time in front of the screen, whether it's a television, cell phone or computer screen? Too much screen time causes major over-stimulation and over-excitement of the brain in most people, which leads to stress, anxiety, trouble sleeping, chronic fatigue and exhaustion, depression and even nausea. I do experience electromagnetic sensitivity on a regular basis when I spend prolonged periods of time in front of the screen. It leads me to feeling anxious, drained, exhausted and very nauseated. In addition, I can only hold my cell phone for short periods of time otherwise my hands become numb and weak. I nearly fainted a few times when I visited the electronic departments of large stores where I felt dizzy and nauseated after only a short time. I managed to get outside as quickly as I could and find a patch of nature to re-balance my energy and remove the toxic overdose of electromagnetic waves I had received, which cured me promptly every time. Needless to say, I no longer visit those places.

Other sources of debilitating electromagnetic radiation impacting our body negatively on measurable or non-measurable levels include the microwave oven, overhead power lines, cell phone towers, 5G technology as well as wireless technology such as wifi and blue tooth headphones. Animals are also affected and often to a greater level due to their smaller body size. Indeed, many birds, bees and other insects have died from electromagnetic radiation from power lines and cell towers, which disrupt the magnetic "compass" that many migrating birds and insects use. They can also disorient mammals and disrupt plant metabolism, leading to the decline of nature. Nature, insects, wild and domestic animals as well as humans (whether they are aware or not) are all electro-sensitive, meaning that they are impacted by electromagnetic waves. Manmade lights that remain bright all night also sadly disorient nocturnal animals and insects. Light pollution has become a big problem in developed countries and is not only harmful but wasteful as well.

In order to make the best and wisest decisions in life for maximum mind, body and soul benefits including balance, harmony and Oneness, we need to enhance our intuition (our body is the best dowsing tool ever) in all aspects of our life.

RECEIVE INFORMATION: At all times remain aware, open and receptive to subtle energetic messages from anyone you meet (humans, animals or nature). It may take the form of words or sentences you HEAR in your head; you may SEE images or movies play in your head; you may FEEL sick, happy, sad or any other emotions that are speaking to you and guiding you; you may all of a sudden KNOW some information or answers you were looking for; you may TASTE or SMELL something that is linked to a message of guidance. You or your animals may get hurt as we discussed before or your animal's bad behavior may be a form of communication, like the canine Dakota who clearly stated he did not want to share his territory by urinating in the house twice, each time after his owners took him to visit with a kitten they were considering adopting.

SEND INFORMATION: To the soul of any human or animal you wish to help, also to communicate with nature and the Universe, which is all done the same way, by focusing on a mental image, or feeling the emotions to send someone, for example safety, love or healing. You can picture in your head what you would like your loved one to do. It is important to focus on the things you want to happen, as opposed to picturing the behavior or problem you don't want. You may also send a question with words in your head or by feeling an emotion like are you jealous? Scared? Lonely? Feeling rejected? Everything can be done either in the physical presence or the absence of a loved one. Even if our loved one is having surgery, is in a coma or in heaven, communication remains the same.

Remember to ask permission first, with love and respect of others' boundaries (out loud or in your head if you can't talk to the other being, and feel for the answer), to make sure it is your place to communicate before you bridge your energies. You may then picture in your head a beautiful bright shining bridge of white light between you and the other being or you can see both of you in a healing, loving and pure white cloud together. Make sure you feel welcome.

To help you focus and bridge your energies, you can look at a picture of the one you wish to communicate with. You can scan it with your hand or your mind by focusing on each body part, one at the time, and feel for heaviness or sickness. You can go one step further and truly become one with your loved one by pretending to enter his body and be him to feel what he feels, to see what he sees and gain his perception on life and the challenges he faces. This can however be very draining emotionally and physically so one must be careful to completely exit out of the body and separate your energies afterwards. You can read more about animal communication in Amelia Kinkade's book, *The Language of Miracles*.

When you get lonely, scared or feeling the pressure to be perfect, wrap yourself in a bubble of white light and protection where you feel safe and loved. Call upon your Family Unit, the Universe, your higher powers whether it is God, Fairies, Nature, Angels, Spirit Animals or deceased loved ones, humans or animals. Remember that no one is perfect; we are all forever students in the school of life. Drop the burden and pressure of being alive and needing to fix the place, it won't be a perfect ride and you won't save the world. Respect your vital boundaries and ask yourself how you can best help the person or animal you have attracted today on your path. Give them the best of yourself, give them your love and support, always keep the magic alive by making them feel special, valued and showing them that their life matters. Then, give yourself a hug and let go of the results. Whatever happens was how it had to happen. Hug yourself again and remember how beautiful you are. Remember who you are, your song, your dance, your place and your soul's purpose on Earth.

Be the teacher for others you wish you had. Be a leader simply by preaching by example. As you grow on your evolutionary journey, you will re-awaken the sensitive and compassionate nature that you were born with. You will become more upset at the world's injustices and greatly feel the pain of others and of the world, which is extremely overwhelming.

How can you deal with it? First, see it as a gift and not a curse. You don't want to go back to your old numb ways. Second, focus on turning the pain you see into action. What can you do to help? Watch the animals relentlessly fighting the good fight along side many compassionate and dedicated human beings to gain justice, dignity and happiness, and join them. How can you become a better teacher for everyone around you? How can you inspire everyone you meet to better care for all animals, all humans, and for our planet? Write three ways to better contribute to your world in your personal life. Write three ways to better contribute to your world at work to make it more meaningful and more fun. Give yourself a pat on the back, you are a better person than you were yesterday. There is so much potential for this world to become a kind, peaceful and loving place.

In order not to feel overwhelmed, I write down all the ideas and actions I want to take. I let my imagination run wild during those brainstorming moments because there is no limit as to what can be accomplished, and every completed action starts with a vision. I then focus on one baby step at the time, always listening with my heart to the signs of guidance to make sure it is my place to pursue this or that idea. I follow the energy flow to feel what idea needs to take priority. It sometimes takes years for an idea to become the priority, but I trust the Universe that the timing will become right for each one and that my role to play in accomplishing them will become clear, all in good time. It is amazing how the Universe doesn't forget. Many times I have seen the window finally open for an idea to take the forefront of my life and for my time to be freed so I can dedicate myself to making it come true. We must trust the process.

Here are a few additional questions I find extremely important for everybody of all ages to answer (with our brain and our heart), and to keep re-visiting throughout our earthly journey to help us stay on track of fulfilling our incarnation and living our best life. The goal of life is to be the best version of ourselves possible and live the life of an exemplary human being, which means with compassion, balance and sustainability.

- You are in Heaven looking down at our world, what does our planet and its living creatures, animals and humans, need most?
- Imagine you just died and you are reviewing the movie of your life, what do you see? How did you make others feel, animals and humans? What makes you feel sad? What do you wish you had done better? What are your regrets? What do you miss the most? What makes you happy? What are you proud of yourself for? What do you love about yourself?
- Why did you want to come here on Earth? What do you want to learn or accomplish before you die? What do you and your pet live for?
- Today is your last day on Earth, what do you want to change in your life to feel happier and more accomplished, so you can die knowing you gave it your all? The answer should be nothing.
- If today is your last day, how do you want to spend it?
- If you only have two weeks to live, what are your priorities in life?
- If you only have one year to live, what do you want to do to make yourself happy?
- If the world were perfect, what would you do with yourself? Whether the world is perfect or not, you can only accomplish so much and you still need to take care of yourself, so you can then help others. Your life goal should be to become the best person you can be and

share what you have learned with others. This means that no matter how the rest of the world is, perfect or not, your job is the same: to become fulfilled, to thrive and to achieve balance.

This powerful exercise helps you realize what you need to focus on today to stay on your life path so that you have no regrets when you die. Great news, you can change anything in your life to make it the way you want it. Dare taking a leap into a new and better life, I see all your potential bursting to come out. There is no better time to start than today. Imagine that there are no obstacles on your path and you can accomplish everything you want, what do you want to do? What would you do if you knew you couldn't fail? Do it now. Create your life vision statement by describing in a few sentences or a few paragraphs what is important to you and how you want to live. Claim your life, dare to live and light up the world!

Chapter 11

The circle of life

"Take care of Nature and Nature will take care of you". When any major natural disaster strikes, I always wonder why. It brings me back to a similar question to which we have already found an answer: why do we get sick? Balance was and is once again at the top of the list. Nature's goal is to remain in balance and as we said before, Nature teaches us balance.

What if the Earth is like our body and humans are like a disease attacking the Earth? The Earth will try to fight and get rid of it to regain balance. Humans have definitely forgotten balance and have been behaving like a very invasive disease, spreading far and wide, taking over the body of the Earth, which has become overwhelmed, sick and out of balance.

However, Nature won't die without a fight. Nature strikes against humans on a regular basis, maybe each strike is a warning to live more in balance, maybe the strikes will get more and more violent, kill more and more people, and result in the extinction of the human race if humans don't listen and learn fast. When Mother Nature sends humans a virus forcing everyone to stay home, she breathes with relief. The pollution stops. The skies and the waters return to blue. The wild animals catch their breath as well and take back their territory by visiting beaches, rivers and cities.

Scientists believe that since the beginning of times, most pandemics that have decimated human populations have been caused by humans getting too close to animals. From domesticating and farming animals since ancient times, to modern days where we are destroying their habitats and encroaching on their territory, both have led to close contact and animals sharing their viruses and bacteria with humans. Furthermore, our self-destruction and self-extinction continues with our excessive airplane use facilitating the transmission of contagious diseases all around the world at record speed, combined with our overly dense population creating a human chain through which the virus propagates quickly and effectively. The human race is its own worst enemy.

If we had asked everyone to stay home to save the Earth, most would not have cared. Humans are motivated by what they choose to see. Avoiding pain for themselves and gaining pleasure are the two biggest motivators, and both are directly influenced by the reality and the fears one chooses to create and focus on. Losing their own life to a virus is a big enough motivation for most. Most people, however, still don't realize that in order to save ourselves, we first need to save the Earth. Then after a short while of being confined at home, many people choose to shift their focus onto a new fear, the fear of losing too much money by staying home and how detrimental it will be to me, me, me… They never ask how the Earth is doing because they take her for granted. Most people don't fear losing the Earth and her rich resources. Most people are ready to get back to their old routine of destruction and feelings of entitlement as if we were king of the mountain and the Earth with her endless resources is our slave.

A very contagious virus targeting the entire human population brings humility, gratitude and vulnerability. It pulls the rug out from under our feet and it destabilizes us. It forces us to slow down and rethink how fragile life and the whole world truly are. It makes us question what life is about and how simple it can and should be. We call society the rat race but humans have taken it to a whole other level. The human race is by far the worst kind of race, in both senses of the word. When we are forced to stop all non-essential activities (or non-sense activities?), the world comes to a halt. What more can one need beside clean air, water, sun, food, shelter, love and medical care? Natural crises give us an incredible chance to wake up from our complacent and excessive state, re-adjust, step up, get our priorities straight, and dare to think outside of the box to create healthier and higher standards of what we consider normal in society. Natural crises give us an incredible opportunity to become better humans.

How much of the non-essential stuff do we need? How much is that non-essential stuff helping Nature, or how much is it harming Nature? What have humans done to the Earth? Those natural crises remind us that we should always fear and respect Nature. Nature can wipe the human race out very quickly. Who is really essential to the Earth? Animals are, like bees, but not humans, so the Earth doesn't care if we don't survive. If we kill Nature, we kill ourselves. By helping Nature, we help ourselves. That should always be everyone's primary focus. It is not too late to ask Mother Nature for forgiveness and become minimalist, which means living with less stuff. Tell her how sorry you are for your clueless, selfish and destructive behavior. Let's stop wasting our time, our energy and our life with non-sense distractions and let's use our time, energy and life to educate ourselves and the next generations about critical topics to save the Earth and ourselves. Let's live a meaningful life. Thank Mother Nature for everything she gives you so generously. Tell her and, most importantly, show her how much you love her and value her by improving your behavior. Hug her by laying down on the grass and practice grounding or earthing, as previously discussed. Become One with Mother Nature and learn to work as a team. Most importantly, always fear losing her.

Should we be afraid of death? No, because death is inevitable. However, we should be afraid of dying separated from Mother

Nature, unfulfilled in that complacent, lost and numb mental and emotional state dictated by a sick society. We should also be afraid of dying at the wrong time. How do we prevent that? By making sure we become aware, awake, and have no regret or guilt in the decisions we make. Our decisions should be made for the right reasons, which are to find fulfillment, live on purpose and feed our soul. Not for greed, power or to fuel our ego. We should also make sure that we follow guidance from Mother Nature as well as our intuition to find our place everyday. Our place can change rapidly. Where is my place today; where do I belong to serve the Universe, for the greater good of our world? Is it at home, at work, working on this or that project or relaxing and playing with the animals, or doing volunteer work? When you are in your place, doing what you are meant to be doing and you die, that was the right time to die. Many people will choose to sacrifice themselves (because it is the place they chose to fulfill their incarnation subconsciously) to help our world rise to a new level of consciousness during natural disasters, including victims, paramedics and other first responders.

By listening to our three brains at all times, we will make the best decisions that are in our control: the rational brain in our head for critical thinking, problem solving and analysis; the emotional brain in our heart to follow our passions and stay true to who we are; the intuitive brain in our gut to feel if a decision is right or not for us, also for courage and risk-taking.

Furthermore, there are many ways to boost our immune system and help prevent or fight diseases. First, common sense dictates that social distancing and washing our hands often will help prevent contraction of contagious diseases. The next best way is definitely fulfillment. When we live on purpose, work on purpose, feed our soul and shine our brightest by sharing all of our gifts with the world, when our heart, mind and body vibrate pure happiness and we are comfortable with who we are and our incarnation purpose, when we are unleashing all that we are and feeling valued and empowered, our immune system is at its best.

In addition, sleeping well, exercising, eating healthy foods, drinking a lot of water, spending time in nature, getting sun vitamin, limiting fear and stress (we want just enough to motivate us to be at our best, awake, in a high level state of awareness, not too much that it will weaken our immune system), taking life one day at a time, feeling grateful, laughing a lot, hugging someone (healthy animal or human), and sharing love will raise our energy level and make our mind and body feel alive. Singing, playing music, dancing, and doing the things we love also stimulate our body to release good hormones and fortify our immune system (same for our animals). Lastly, one of the most important ways to strengthen our immune system is by hugging our own self. Self-love saves us. Self-love is remembering that you came to this world alone and that you will leave it alone. Therefore, be comfortable being with yourself and taking good care of yourself. Discover your loner power.

In Chinese medicine, each organ has a sound: ee for brain health, sahn for lungs, chee for liver. Many cultures still use bells, chimes, bowls, drums and chanting in ceremony to uplift and purify the energy. A healthy body is when each cell of each organ creates a resonance in harmony with the whole being. When an energy blockage occurs, the ill organ stops vibrating at a healthy frequency. Sound therapy helps release blockages in the body.

I have brushed against a few natural disasters including 9/11/2001 when I took the subway in the World Trade Center one hour before it crumbled. I also missed a drive-by shooting by five hours in Las Vegas as well as a mass shooting at a local political event by two hours. Why did I not die? Why not me? I believe it was not part of my incarnation plan. Furthermore, the law of attraction and karma are, once again, always ready to give us back what we put out in the world. The more we take care of Mother Nature by saving insects, gardening, planting trees, not wasting foods, adopting a child or an animal instead of breeding, protecting spider webs, sparingly using the entire roll of toilet paper (or better even is using a bidet), adopting a vegan, eco-friendly and zero-waste lifestyle, limiting pollution by traveling less, picking up others' litter, saving resources by reusing, recycling and saying no to excessive consumerism, the more we inject healing energy into the web of life and into our body.

Nature in return sends it back by taking care of us, protecting us and loving us through, for example, sending us a beautiful and natural pond to swim in, having dragonflies land on our hands and saving our life during natural disasters. I can honestly and proudly say that my life has not changed much at all because of COVID-19. Caring for nature and social distancing have always made more sense to me as a way to escape the exhausting turmoil caused by the human race.

By taking life simply, one day at a time like the animals do, we develop resilience and adaptability. We learn to become a team with Mother Nature. We learn to feel stable even during one of the most unstable times in history. Living each day like you could get a virus and die gives you clarity. Living each day like it is your last day makes your life the most meaningful. Don't wait for anyone but yourself to be proud of what you are accomplishing. Don't wait for anyone but Mother Earth to praise you and compliment you. Nature will send you her blessings, believe me. Become a part of something bigger than yourself. You need the Earth and the Earth needs you. Gratitude is the attitude. Be grateful for the pure water you drink, the pure air you breathe. Be grateful for the lush forests and sparkling waters you have seen in your lifetime. Save the Earth, save yourself! Be Oneness, Be Greatness!

Please find a piece of paper you can reuse (or pick a blank page from this book) and write down your answers to these very important questions:

Are you listening to Mother Nature talking to you? Are you Oneness with your environment? Are you asking permission before you take anything from Nature? Do you only take what is necessary to survive? Do you thank her? How can you live more in harmony and balance with your world, Nature and its living creatures? Do you walk the Earth with respect, love and compassion? Have you ever visited your local landfill where waste materials are magically disposed of? If not, please arrange to take a eye opening field trip as soon as possible to see how unmagical it is and how mindful we should be about throwing away anything in the garbage, it will forever change you for the better. How did you generously help another living creature lately? How did you make this creature feel? How did it make you feel? How can you become an inspiration and example for others to follow? How can you give back to Nature more than you take from Nature? Do you attract natural disasters, a house fire, freak accidents, snakes and spiders? Make a list and try to figure out why you attracted them. Do you crush every single spider, ant or fly you see? Or maybe kill weeds or uproots plants or cactus that you don't like? Do you waste water? Maybe Mother Nature has been sending you messages that it is time to make a change. You can change your karma now! Take as little as you need, give as much as you can.

Meditation to live in harmony and become One with the web of life:

Welcome to the New World. Close your eyes and open your heart. Take deep breaths and ……… relax.

Let go of all your fears, worries and frustrations. Breathe out all your fears, worries and frustrations. Let go of feeling the pain of the world.

Feel light and free. Trust that in the circle of life, everything happens for the greater good of this world. You are at home in the circle of life. You are safe and loved.

Wholeheartedly put your arms around your shoulders and hug yourself right now while saying: You are worthy of love and happiness "your name", you are beautiful and you matter. Repeat this sentence as many times as you need to feel safe and protected.

See the world around you with new eyes. Feel the peace. We feel safe in the circle of life because all living creatures are united, as One, supporting one another.

Feel the amazing connection between all life forms and the powerful teamwork manifesting.

We are One, our essence has become One, WE are the web of life. Feel your physical body disappearing and fusing with this divine life force all around.

We now are the agile squirrel running up a tree to safety, we are the mindful bird flying food to feed its young, we are the artist spider building its fragile web.

Our mind expands as we watch the miracle of life unfold before our eyes. We are discovering all the magnificent and magical ways Nature manifests herself through all her different creations.

Our soul feels infinite compassion for the fragile web of life that we now want to protect with all that we are. Our body has disappeared, our energy is now deeply connected with Nature, Mother Earth, Father sky and all forms of life, WE are One.

We are the ants working diligently in unison; we are the lions roaring loudly, claiming their presence, protecting the land and standing up strong for one another; we are the fish living in balance in their ecosystem; we are the elephants joining forces in sharing motherly knowledge, wisdom and critical thinking through generations; we are the trees breathing deeply as we are the lungs of our beautiful planet; we are the clear and clean water running through the rivers as we are the veins of our wonderful home called Earth.

Listen and watch Nature, the animals, the plants and the insects expressing themselves, fulfilling their powerful incarnation, being the best they can be. When we help them thrive, we help ourselves achieve balance and prosperity.

Feel the whole animal kingdom hugging you as you are in the center of the circle of life. Feel the pure white blanket of light, love and gratitude animals are wrapping you in, thanking you for your care, respect, compassion and value for all life forms. Like them, you are a teacher of kindness and the world needs you.

You are the sun and you radiate your peace, your love and your guidance onto others. You teach everyone to be mindful of their every action to protect our resources, to live simply and to achieve zero waste. Together we not only survive but we thrive. Be Oneness, Be Greatness! Xxx

Chapter 12

The New and Healthier Health Care System for Both Animals and People

The current health care system for both animals and humans needs a heart. The goal of medicine is to cure and to not torture because of greed, for money or because we are afraid of death. As long as there is life on Earth, there is a chance to fix the currently sick medical system. For that, our "industry" desperately needs good leaders. The for-profit system created by the modern world is shameful and flagrantly unacceptable. Caring so much about it hurts but I can't stop caring. I don't want to stop caring about all of the animal and human lives that our sick health care system has failed and continues to fail everyday. Too many animals and people have had their lives stolen from them. Society has failed them terribly and is continuing to do so.

Every single decision made by receptionists, nurses, doctors, big pharmaceutical companies and the government must have the patient's best interest at heart. The goal must not be to make money, sell medications, keep patients sick, prolong suffering or perform unnecessary tests or procedures because it means more money coming in. Sadly, too often, a patient doesn't get the help needed when there is no money to be made. This is a tragedy and a crime against humanity. It is a crime against humanity when lives are at stake and we disregard them as having no value because making money is more important. How much is a life worth? Why aren't all lives worth the same?

Or are they? Soldiers and military dogs who give their lives on the battlefield had better die for a good reason, not for an unjustified war motivated by greed and power. War victims, civilians and wounded soldiers better be emotionally and physically well cared for. Everyone better show compassion, humility, support and respect towards others' pain and sacrifice. When will everyone care enough?

For as long as the world has existed rivalry has been present, which is obviously needed for basic survival. Sadly, we haven't evolved any and have even regressed. Most humans have taken competition to a sick extreme. From competing among ourselves starting at a younger and younger age (children stealing toys from one another, fighting, bullying and killing without remorse, also taking school sports to a sick obsession and causing many teenagers to suffer life-long emotional and physical injuries), to adults bullying and crushing each other at work, bosses and world leaders pushing workers to their ultimate mental and physical exhaustion and even death, all is done in the name of greed and power.

How can we believe this is sane, normal or acceptable? How can so many people believe that their lives are worth more than other human lives, worth more than the animal lives that they kill to eat and wear? Worth more than the animal lives that they use to make money via forced competing, forced breeding then cruelly tearing babies away from their mothers to sell or kill and make more money, forced animal testing which has also been taken to a cruel extreme in the name of money? Worth more than the insects they crush without any remorse, worth more than the survival of their home planet that they destroy without care?

The majority of us haven't figured out that compassion and team effort allow us to go further than where we can go alone. Together we can move mountains that were too heavy for any single person. Our differences are our strengths for balance and sustainability. Balance is once again the key. Healthy competition is good and must remain, but we should mainly compete with ourselves to push ourselves to the maximum of our abilities and potential, and therefore live our best life, which benefits not just ourselves but our community and our world.

Once again, the answer is simple and full of common sense: Mother Nature teaches us that extremes are rarely good, life is not black or white, life is not yes or no. Often the answer is where balance is, somewhere in the middle, sometimes yes, sometimes no. This concept leads the way in medicine. Vaccines, just like most medications, are sometimes good and sometimes bad. Abortion is sometimes right, sometimes not. Same thing with euthanasia, the situation and timing must be right.

The new and healthier health care system needed for animals and people is a not-for-profit system that prioritizes patient care and ending suffering. Ending suffering means healing and saving lives when they can be saved, but it also means facilitating a death with dignity when it has become the best option for the animal or human patient. Even when we are mindful to preserve the good quality of life a patient has, to do no harm and to not make things worse, we don't always succeed at helping and nature sometimes takes its course. When we agree to dispense even the mildest medication, we alter the course of nature. Therefore, it is only fair to go all the way and have euthanasia as an option to end suffering when all else has failed.

In this new and healthier health care system, there is no medical torture and no medical neglect. Every being gets the help they need and deserve. Each patient's family also gets the support and education they need and deserve. No one dies of starvation or treatable injuries due to lack of care, funds or resources. No one wrongfully stays alive when there is no more quality of life. Once again, let's remember that everyone who lives will also die.

Compassionate patient care means gentleness in all our manipulations (including removing a simple catheter tape from a leg or an arm). Dogs and cats have died from the stress of a nail trim or a grooming session, and I have witnessed a dog having a seizure from the anticipation of pain every time she would walk into the hospital. Be gentle and creative in everything you do, such as administering oral medication. Give a water chaser afterwards to help the pill get swallowed. Give adequate medication to control pain; do not over-vaccinate; shave hair to facilitate blood draw; choose wisely which procedures should be done at home or at the hospital to reduce stress, which is unique for each patient; talk to your patients often and refer to them by their name, not their disease; go slow, be patient, be helpful and not reckless. Healing often takes time.

Dentists and eye doctors join the rest of the doctors in this new not-for-profit health care system that takes care of the whole body and in which all costs are greatly reduced, such as costs of services, medications as well as medical schooling, with ceiling caps for drug and diagnostic equipment manufacturing companies. Health is not a luxury but a vital need. No medical school should be for profit, which is a huge failure towards the next generation. In this new system, in exchange for cheaper and affordable schooling, doctors receive a smaller salary but have none to minimal debts, and are much happier and fulfilled about the service they provide to their community.

Most doctors desperately want job satisfaction and a good quality of life. Too many doctors unfortunately self-prescribe anti-depressants and hate their job. They value and crave the sacred bond with their patients, they want to spend quality time with them and build a relationship, they want to help them more. They do not want to fill out stacks of insurance papers and be told how to practice medicine by heartless insurance companies. We don't need a middleman ruining the doctor-patient relationship.

There is no more need for health insurance that distracts doctors from treating their patients the way they feel is right and fair in the new health care system. Everyone pays for the services they get at affordable prices. Government help is available with discounts to people who qualify, called charity, and every citizen gets government help as well in case of a catastrophic event (like COVID-19, wildfire or hurricane), in exchange for paying federal taxes. Making health care completely free has disadvantages, the biggest being that too many people will abuse and clog the system, hurting the patients who truly need to be cared for. No country in the world has the resources to perform an MRI on every patient. Triage and common sense from the medical team is mandatory to practice smart and sustainable medicine. Sadly, the current medical system is also extremely wasteful of medications and supplies, which must stop immediately.

Moreover, people tend to forget the value of free services and become easily unappreciative and demanding, which escalates quickly to chaos in a large, modern society. There is more medical torture when health care is free (or when people have money to afford medical care) and the medical team must lead the way to practicing balanced and fair medicine no matter what the situation is, which means using critical thinking and common sense to perform only the necessary tests and treatments sick patients need in order to preserve resources and keep the patient's dignity.

In the new system, paying for services out of pocket helps people be responsible and take better care of themselves, and thus avoid becoming sick in the first place. It motivates them to be involved in their own care and health to avoid medical expenses. Classes are held to inform, educate and discuss relevant health topics of all kinds (including how alcohol and cigarettes ruin lives; how feeding horses at ground level, like in the wild, is healthier; how high heel shoes are bad for the feet and the whole posture; the pros and cons of cultural circumcision; how to pick the best time and age for sterilization surgery for each animal to prevent physical, psychological and emotional negative impact; and how our modern houses often severely injure our beloved pets with their slippery floors and large glass windows and doors).

The greatest medicine of all is to teach and empower people how not to need it, and how to heal themselves and their animals. People who have the means are encouraged to donate money to a special fund to help other animal and human patients in need. Their donation is tax deductible. Most importantly, this makes wealthy people feel good about helping less fortunate fellow humans and animals heal and live. Communities could encourage compassionate bonding between donors and recipients of funds by putting together "We are saving lives" events and opportunities for them to meet and grow by getting to know each other's situation. Recipients are encouraged to give back to society in any way they can, by volunteering their time to visit lonely patients in nursing homes or shelter animals for example, which brings a lot of comfort and gratification to everyone involved. Everyone is good at something and can contribute to society.

Transparency is at the forefront in the new and healthier health care system. The population knows what is happening behind closed doors. Research projects involving animals are accessible to the public and everyone gets to vote on them. There is democracy of what is acceptable and what is not tolerated. People become sensitized and woken up, as opposed to being made callous and numb to what's happening like it is in the current system. A not-for-profit medical system would greatly reduce animal testing, which is for the most part senseless, wasteful and cruel for both cosmetic and medical reasons. We must get back in touch with reality, live life with no blinders, and hopefully reach a point of zero testing all together.

We can prevent torture of billions of animals that are used for testing to try to find cures to many diseases caused by eating animals in the first place. We have already discussed all the health benefits of adopting a vegan diet, processing our emotions and having a balanced lifestyle. There are many owned pets as well as people battling illnesses such as chronic pain, seizures and cancer, who would voluntarily participate in research projects as their last resort, knowing that they can be euthanized if their condition worsens, and by doing so reduce the need to involve healthy animals. We must allow any and all proven and promising alternative methods of healing to be shared with patients, which will help further reduce the need for laboratory animals. Fortunately, science has finally proven how powerful the mind is by recognizing the healing placebo effect of positive emotions as well as the harmful nocebo effect of negative emotions. Let's continue to find and share new ways to heal!

In addition, we need to limit the duration of testing and allow adoption of laboratory animals able to have a good life and to receive love, which is only fair after the painful tests we have put them through. We must dedicate at least one day per year, but ideally one day a month, to recognize the lives of those who have died for us and our pets, to show our gratitude towards them, and to honor their pain and suffering. We must take pride in what we are doing, in what the human race is doing, and not be satisfied with mediocrity. We must have moral integrity and a clear conscience. Our health care system and our whole world will thrive when it has a heart.

Chapter 13

Unite, Inspire & Empower

1. Your only competition is with yourself to be a better person today than you were yesterday.
2. Do you have a problem for every solution or a solution for every problem?
3. Your worth is calculated by who you are, not what you have. Your worth is calculated by what you do with what you have. Are you helping our world or hurting it?
4. The world needs "human change", which would fix everything. Humans must change and become transparent in everything they do. Decency and accountability will save the human race. Be a good human.
5. Stay light and be the light. Light up the world! Be the teacher and leader the world needs. Never miss an opportunity to educate others and to show the way with patience and compassion.
6. Live each day like it's your first day on Earth and like it's your last day on Earth. What are the causes that you find worth fighting for? Living for? Dying for?
7. Quality of life over quantity. Quality of friends over quantity. Quality of death is as important as quality of life.
8. Mistakes and failures are often blessings in disguise. Enjoy navigating on the ocean of life with your loved ones. Be grateful for just being with them and accompanying one

another. Everyone is on their unique journey of figuring things out for themselves. You can't save others from making mistakes or taking wrong turns, those lessons are rich in teachings. Just be there to hold their hand and have your hand held while making them.

9. Common sense is sadly uncommon.
10. If it bugs you emotionally, it will bug you physically. We hurt the way we are.
11. Take time to breathe, to chew, to laugh, to hug yourself, and to be. Take time to live before you die. Money can't buy time, use yours wisely.
12. Your biggest life battle is with yourself so get out of your own way and don't sabotage yourself. The sooner you face and slay your inner demons, the better your life will be. Only you can do it, only you can free and save yourself.
13. The more Zen we are, the more Zen animals and people around us will be. Be the best version of yourself, be the best you can be and your pet will be the same. When we live together, we become like one another.
14. Stop trying to fit in the box you don't want to fit in. Dare being YOUR self, live your life YOUR way! Honor your Essence. You were born to stand out.
15. Life is a series of baby steps, small choices and small actions. Constant small changes (and therefore challenges) are necessary for growth and evolution. Be brave and take life one small step at the time.
16. Live your life like you are on the Titanic, because you are. Make the best of your voyage on Earth before it ends.
17. Hold a "celebration of life" party instead of funerals, and invite your dying loved one to attend before he or she dies, animal or human.

18. You may disappoint others, but don't disappoint yourself. Don't ever let yourself down.
19. You are not crazy, you are a visionary. Always remember who you are at your core.
20. Choose not to worry and to be happy. All is well. Life is here and now.
21. You are who you think you are. Life is what you think it is. Everyone creates his own perception and reality. Heaven and Hell are on Earth.
22. When you feel lost in life, watch what the animals do and copy; ask for guidance and follow Mother Nature and the Universe's energy flow; keep it simple.
23. We can't eat or breathe money. Let's remember life's priorities.
24. Write your own life story, only YOU decide who you are. Love yourself enough to set boundaries and protect yourself. Make your dreams come true. Never give up on yourself.
25. Believe in yourself and in your dreams when no one else does. Be your best friend and your biggest fan always!
26. Be like a mountain no one can shake or destabilize. Resist the strongest winds and storms.
27. Save your energy for what is truly important in life, which does not include gossiping, bullying, judging, complaining or showing off. Use your energy to feed your soul, to fulfill yourself and to show others the loving and compassionate way towards themselves and towards others. Focus your energy where you will create great things.
28. Do the right thing because karma is always watching.
29. Don't pollute with your speech. Speak less, mean more and teach always. Silent power.

30. I value you, I value your life, I value your suffering and you matter.
31. What is right for you is not necessarily right for me.
32. Choose whatever religion inspires you to do good around you. Make everything you do, each small action, meaningful and impactful.
33. Security and safety seem to be an illusion in a chaotic world where evolution is the goal and changes are constant. However, we can learn to feel safe and stable even through ever-changing times.
34. Happiness is within. Choose to be happy. Create your own magic in your happy bubble, and share it with everyone else! Laughter is the shortest distance between two people.
35. When others tell you that what you want to do is impossible to achieve, it's because they can't, but YOU can.
36. If I erase the mistakes from my past, I erase the great person I have become because of them.
37. Gratitude is the attitude. Don't be sad for what the world is not, be grateful for all its beauties. Don't be sad when something is over, be glad it happened. Your life is someone else's dream.
38. Follow your passions and your vision, and you will never get lost. Your heart knows the way. When we love what we do, we forget to be scared of doing it, or scared of what others will think, or scared of failing. Don't be afraid of failure, be afraid of not doing the things you really love and want to do. Your goals must be greater than your fears. To overcome fear, sometimes you must close your eyes and just go for it!
39. Plant seeds and accept that you might not be there to see the trees grow, but they will.

40. Don't worry about not making a difference because we all make a difference. Worry about making a positive difference.
41. Make sure all your relationships with animals and humans are healing and freeing, as opposed to toxic and limiting. Each animal and human needs space to themselves.
42. Don't be afraid of losing people. Be afraid of losing yourself trying to please everyone around you. Meet your own needs first and keep your dreams alive.
43. Your life is unique, there was never anyone else like you before and there will never be anyone else like you after you die. Don't blend in. Shine your brightest!
44. Exist kindly. Speak kind words only.
45. You were born alone and you will die alone. Learn to be comfortable and happy in your company. You are the only person you will be with your whole life.
46. The best thing about having regrets is that it means we have grown. We now know better and we will do better. It's not over until you are dead. Get back on your feet and try again.
47. Thank you for making the world a better place with your smile, kindness, love and happiness. The world needs love. Everyone needs love and love is all we need. Smile and hug often.
48. You are what you eat, and you should eat in accordance with who you are.
49. No one can take away your inner peace unless you let them.
50. The answer is often: TOGETHER
51. Fight for what you believe in no matter what anyone says. Don't go numb, be the voice of the voiceless, be a leader, do or die.
52. Find the one matching your crazy to share life with. Be crazy, it is the only way to stay sane!

53. Good or bad, others remember how you made them feel. Make animals and people you meet feel the best they have ever felt!
54. Be good, be caring, be loving, be genuine. Live so that when others think of integrity and authenticity, they think of you. Be the leader you are looking for.
55. Life won't be perfect. It has cracks filled with learning opportunities and growth. Things you do and actions you take might not be perfect either, but most of the time they will be enough to continue your advancement on your beautiful path of self-achievement. Enjoy your journey of life and make it perfectly imperfect.
56. If your actions inspire others to dream more, learn more, do more and become more, you are a leader. – John Quincy Adams
57. Live simply so that others may simply live. – Mahatma Gandhi
58. I never fail, either I succeed, or I learn. – Nelson Mandela
59. If you wanna do something, you'll find a way. If you don't, you'll find an excuse. – Jim Rohn
60. People crazy enough to think they can change the world are the ones who do. – Steve Jobs
61. Logic will get you from A to B. Imagination will take you everywhere. – Albert Einstein
62. It is no measure of good health to be well adjusted to a profoundly sick society. – Jiddu Krishnamurti
63. Normal is an illusion. What is normal for the spider is chaos for the fly. – Morticia Addams
64. Everybody is a genius. But if you judge a fish by its ability to climb a tree, it will live its whole life believing that it is stupid. – Albert Einstein

65. The true measure of any society can be found in how it treats its most vulnerable members. – Mahatma Gandhi
66. Great minds discuss ideas, average minds discuss events and small minds discuss people. – Eleanor Roosevelt
67. Winners are not people who never fail but people who never quit. – Ed Cole
68. There is always a cloud in the sky and a ray of sunshine, you decide which one you want to focus on.
69. "I love you, I'm sorry, Forgive me, Thank you" are powerful words to heal our relationships. Also powerful are: "I love me, I forgive me, I value me, I thank me, I hug me, I am free".
70. You are more powerful than you know. Use your three brains at all times to make your best decisions: head, heart and gut.
71. Remember that we each see life through a very unique pair of glasses, based on our life experiences, good and bad. Be tolerant and compassionate. Try to understand why someone's views and opinions are different.
72. Take pride in what you do, give it your 100% no matter what it is.
73. All that matters in the end is my own opinion of myself. Did I hold myself to the high standards I wish everyone else had? Don't wait for others to compliment you. Don't lower your expectations to meet others' low standards. Be proud of what you have accomplished. Praise yourself and only try to impress yourself.
74. Better to gift a loved one with euthanasia one day too early than one day too late.
75. Be noble in all your actions no matters what others do. You must be able to live with yourself.
76. Listen to your pet when he or she doesn't like a new friend of yours. Your pet is often a better judge of character than you

are and may save you a lot of time, energy and heartache if you follow his or her advice of not trusting someone.

77. The one who stops learning stops living. The one who stops hoping, dreaming and believing in a brighter tomorrow starts dying. Remain curious about life and want more from life always.
78. When I feel sad and powerless, I speak to the soul of the one I feel the pain of, the one I wish I could help and say: "Thank you for giving your life to elevate the consciousness of our world/ to awaken your family's awareness and compassion. Thank you for helping your family/ our world grow. I wish I could do more to help you. Your suffering and death were not in vain. I value your sacrifice, I value your being, I value your life, I love you".
79. We all have the same life lessons to learn because the goal of life is the same for all: balance.
80. Love like you have never been hurt, live like you have never been disappointed. There are a few decent people out there worth meeting who can help us make our dreams come true.
81. The art of living: knowing when to let go and when to hang on.
82. In the end, only three things matter: how much you loved, how gently you lived, and how gracefully you let go of things not meant for you. – Buddha
83. The secret of making dreams come true can be summarized in 4 Cs. They are curiosity, confidence, courage and constancy; and the greatest of all is confidence. – Walt Disney
84. First, think. Second, dream. Third, believe. And finally, dare. – Walt Disney
85. That's the real problem with the world, too many people grow up. – Walt Disney

86. Be more, do less, we are human beings, not human doings.
87. The intention matters more than the results. When you have given everything you could, let go of the results and laugh. Pieces will fall wherever they want to fall and it's now out of your control. It's ok to cry but then remember to laugh some more, and laugh as hard as you can.
88. You vibrate to the level of what you focus on and what you surround yourself with. Is your life energy high or low? Do you feel alive or dead?
89. When you make a promise to your animal or human loved one, keep it. Be true to your word, act on it and don't disappoint.
90. Love and value yourself so you can love and value others.
91. The human body is made of numerous individual cells. Each of them must take care of its own individual needs while performing a specific job, yet working as a team in order to care for the whole being and create a healthy body. The body of planet Earth is made of numerous individual human-cells. Each of them must take care of its own individual needs while performing a different job, yet working as a team in order to care for the whole being and create a healthy planet.
92. Fake it until you become it. Whatever you want in your future, act as if it was already here. We become who we think we are.
93. If you are happy, at peace with yourself and you bring happiness and peace to others, you are on the right path.
94. Achieve zero waste by donating your long hair to a child in need www.wigsforkids.org.
95. Earth doesn't belong to man, man belongs to the Earth. – Chef Seattle

96. The greatest challenge in life is discovering who you are. The second greatest challenge is being happy with what you find. – Oscar Auliq-Ice
97. You never know how strong you are until being strong is your only choice. – Bob Marley
98. Let your smile change the world, but don't let the world change your smile. – Connor Franta
99. Every time I thought I was being rejected from something good, I was actually being re-directed to something better. – Steve Maraboli
100. Don't wish it were easier, wish you were better. Don't wish for fewer problems, wish for more skills. Don't wish for less challenges, wish for more wisdom. – Earl Shoaf
101. The only thing of importance, when we depart, will be the traces of love we have left behind. – Albert Schweitzer
102. The purpose of life is to find your gift, the meaning of life is to give it away. – David Viscott

CONCLUSION

I have accomplished a lot on this journey of life and, as I said before, my goal is to have no regrets when I die. My powerful life experiences have shaped my beliefs and motivated me to explore the most untouched and controversial paths. Animals have supported me and inspired me through it all.

My message to you today is to continue to listen to your intuition and recognize the synchronicity, messages and signs of guidance in your life to prevent bad experiences and attract only good ones. Stay on your true path always. You are powerful!

What is left for me to do? To continue to inspire everyone to live in balance, as One, with the web of life; teach by example; share peace, love and healing with all living creatures I meet (welcome to the family Rocksie, a new life chapter begins!); make everyone feel valued everyday that I have left on this beautiful planet; achieve a zero-waste lifestyle and hug myself daily. What is humanity's life mission? Growing as souls and living in harmony with our planet and its inhabitants; giving more to Mother Earth than we take.

Because of the way the world is going, I have made peace with the fact that I will most likely not live long enough to see the New World the way I have envisioned it (but hopefully I will see it in a different life form if I choose to reincarnate). Until then, I have envisioned a movie to show everyone how much better the world will be when we all decide to listen to the animals and apply their teachings. Animals have never failed me. By following their guidance, we can truly heal our society and our world. If you have movie industry expertise and connections, please help me bring the movie "Animal Teachings" to life.

Together, we are creating the New World! Thank you for sharing your wisdom with others on your path and for lending a caring hand to those in need, great and small. Please continue to thrive, to awaken all your dormant potential and to be the best you can be, the world needs more people like you!

Animals see humans as a reckless and unsustainable species, out of control and out of balance, yet they believe in us. Let's stop failing them and failing ourselves, we can learn from our mistakes and do better. Since animals are the best teachers for a healthy and balanced society in which humans feel supported through this difficult journey of incarnation, we must put them everywhere. Let's empty the animal shelters and re-home these wonderful teachers in our homes, work offices, schools, nursing homes, prisons, rehabilitation centers and homeless shelters. Animals will save us if we follow their guidance!

And scream, when the time is right, live with all of your might… listen to the inspiring rock song "Breathe" written and performed by my husband at www.DFCrock.com, as well as many other empowering ones! Music helps heal.

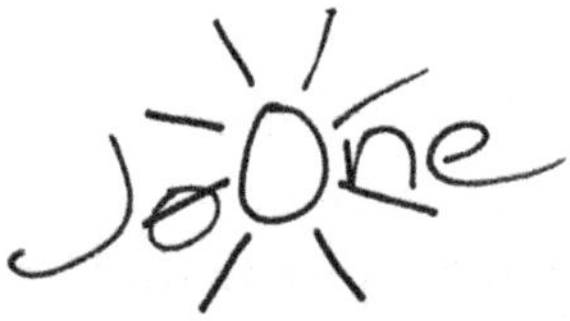

Joanne Lefebvre Connolly, DVM

Contact information: To invite Dr. Joanne to be a guest speaker at your next event or conference, to invite Dr. Joanne to teach your medical and veterinary students, to enroll your hospital (veterinary or human) in receiving personalized teachings and your Hayley's Angels Methods' Hospital Certification,

Contact us: Hayley's Angels Methods
hayleysangels@yahoo.com OR hayleysangels@hotmail.com
www.hayleysangels.com

A HEARTFELT "THANK YOU" FROM GRATEFUL AND ENLIGHTENED READERS OF MY FIRST BOOK

"Animal Teachings from Hayley's Angels Methods"

Could not put book down! I must admit I am not an avid reader. I read Animal Teachings in two days and could not put this book down. Highly recommend this book to animal lovers, people who care about other people, and all people in health care as well as health care providers. Book is written from the heart and experience. Animal Teachings has taught me many things and opened up my eyes! Looking forward to the next book!

From Debbie, Spice & Rocky's mom

The most inspiring book I have ever read! This book is very inspiring! It helps the reader to learn more about themselves and to understand animals in a beautiful way. I felt very good after reading this book, it helped me to realize that my dreams can come true. It increased my understanding of my dogs greatly as well. I highly recommend this book to anyone who likes to feel uplifted.

From Kate Hinner, Tucson AZ

A Soul Searching, Insightful Book! This book helped my husband and I to look at life from perspectives other than what we were used to. Dr. Lefebvre's gift is her ability to be so compassionate and in touch with not only her patients but also their parents and the life around us. Dr. Lefebvre's book encouraged us to think deeply about our own life and its impact on the planet. It gave me ideas on how to improve my interactions with my own patients and also the environment. A must-read for anyone who believes there is more out there. We can all become better citizens of our planet with a little bit of this knowledge. Thank you Dr. Lefebvre.

From Melanie Olson, DVM

Joanne, I truly loved your book and am honored to be mentioned in it. I read it so fast and just like another one of your friends, have to go back with the highlighter now. It's been going on three years since Coco passed away and I still miss him so much. Reading your book was like telling a secret to a friend who really understands. Such a sense of comfort and support. Thank you!!

Brigid Cleary

Dear Joanne, thank you so much for helping us with Zoot and for the nice card. I saw your video and I have been reading your book, which is wonderful. Thank you for doing so much to make the world a better place. Shifting consciousness is very important and something I have been studying myself. However, it has been somewhat depressing and I have been feeling like the problems of this world are just too big for me to do anything about. However, my interaction with you and your book reminded me that even the little things count so I have decided to move towards vegetarianism by giving up beef and pork immediately and then eliminating chicken and seafood in time. I have also changed my dog's diet. Thank you for your personal story and your dedication. Thank you for letting your sweet soul radiate goodness out into the world. In the past 3.5 years we have lost a total of five pets, two parents and one friend, and I had been starting to get very negative, but meeting you renewed my hope.

Thank you so much for that, Melissa Mauzy

Insight into helping your pet and yourself! Working in the veterinary field for years, I have walked out of many exam rooms saying to myself 'I wish this "pet" could really tell me what's going on'. If you could find a way to communicate with your most beloved companion, wouldn't you want to? If your pet was ill and you needed assistance in finding what to do, and conventional medicine couldn't provide that, what would you do? Dr. Joanne Lefebvre, DVM has brought intuitive medicine to light, and is helping pets and people because of it. Although intuitive medicine has been around forever, it has sadly become forgotten by many in our modern society. Thanks to Dr. Lefebvre, everyone can now learn how to awaken their dormant intuition to reach maximum health and happiness, as well as how to express their full potential during their journey on Earth. Dr. Lefebvre is using intuitive medicine in conjunction with conventional medicine to assist in finding the cause of a physical or emotional condition in animals. When combining the two approaches, your pet gets the best results. In this book, Dr. Lefebvre shares some of her communications and success stories during her journey of learning how intuitive medicine wants to use her. It's amazing to read some of these experiences and communications and to truly feel the connection. I highly recommend this book if you want insight into helping your pet and/or yourself, discovering who you and your pet truly are on a soul level, and learning to live your life while staying in tune with your life purpose at all times.

From Lisa Schrope, Certified and Registered Veterinary Technician

Dearest Joanne, thank you so very much for helping our Bridget to leave this world and enter heaven with such ease. We really struggled with trying to save her life and it was a blessing not to struggle with her trying to end it. I have read your book and if everyone felt like you do, no one would have to suffer when ready to leave this world. Thank God for people like you.

It takes a thoughtful individual like you to help others in their time of greatest need.

The Reece family

Thank goodness there was you! Joanne, I don't even know what to say that you probably haven't heard a thousand times already, so I'll just say what I'm feeling and what echoes the many letters you've received from others. I want to thank you so much for helping Maggie cross over. I can't even explain to you how happy I am that one phone call led me to you. This was difficult for us and you helped us with the process and gave us space to say goodbye, and didn't make it feel rushed or uncomfortable. And as trivial as it might seem, it was special to me to see her leave looking so beautiful wrapped up in that pretty pink blanket. I told my husband if she had to leave with anyone, you were the one! Such a loving, kind spirit. What you do and who you are is a HUGE blessing in this world. I could feel that from you, but after I read your book I feel like it confirmed it. What a gift that you shared so much of yourself in your writing. It really gave me a lot to think about as well—not only in dealing with animals, but about life in general. I've been reading the peace exercise at the end of chapter 11. I'm hoping if I read it every morning it will sink in before long!

Thank you so much, Christa

An excellent read and thought-provoking! A must-read for anyone who has pets and/or people they care about! After reading this book you will have a whole new perspective on caring for your animals and advocating for your family and friends when they are ill or in need of medical care. Read with an open mind and know that even if your own philosophies do not align with those of Dr. Lefebvre, you will come away with an improved understanding of your pets and their needs.

From Pam Stabach, Veterinary Hospital Office Manager

Healing the mind, body and soul of animals and of people
Dr. Joanne Lefebvre's new book, "Animal Teachings," forever removed from my mind the false division between what, in our Western culture, are referred to as the scientific and the spiritual domains. Not that she has not admirably distinguished herself in her difficult area of science, Veterinary Medicine; far from it. As an animal doctor, she draws on a vast compendium of solid, detailed, technical knowledge; but Dr. Lefebvre has more than the current science models operating when she strives to cure and care for the animals under her care: it's a deep, intuitive response to a dimension of knowing we simplistically refer to as the spiritual. Tell me of another exceptional veterinarian who not only seeks deep, hidden communication with such creatures as whales, but has the professional courage to say so in a widely published book? In the end, this physician tells us what all the greatest physicians have, through time, always told us: scientific facts belong to the five physical senses and logical rationality; spiritual facts belong to another sense we call intuition and expand through a welcoming, open intelligence determined to heal the whole person, or the whole animal, not just their bodies. Joanne Lefebvre makes ample use of both. Listen deeply to the animals, Dr. Lefebvre counsels us, and you will accomplish things only formerly dreamed of.

From Sammie Ann Wicks, Ph.D., Musicologist, Folklorist, Anthropologist, Americanist, and a grateful client with a grateful kitty.

Biography

Dr. Joanne Lefebvre Connolly is a vegan intuitive veterinarian of the New World and author who empowers all animals and humans to live in balance, as One, with the web of life. She promotes intuitive medicine for the mind, body and soul. "Treat the patient, not just the disease". She inspires families to give themselves and their pets a better quality of life as well as quality of death. "Better living & better dying for all".

Dr. Joanne guides families to tune into their pets, themselves, nature & the Universe to make better, fair and personalized medical and life decisions, prevent diseases and accidents, speed up healing and allow for a peaceful and dignified passing for our loved ones and ourselves. She believes that we can all listen to our intuition and recognize the synchronicity, messages and signs of guidance in our life to prevent bad experiences and attract good ones. We are powerful!

Dr. Joanne grew up in Canada and graduated from the University of Montreal veterinary school in 2001. During her senior year of veterinary school, she completed several externships in highly reputable schools such as Cornell University, Tufts, Colorado and Ohio State Universities. She was one of the very few selected for an internship in small animal medicine, surgery and emergency at Michigan Veterinary Specialists, which she proudly completed. She published a scientific & clinical study in the British Journal of Small Animal Practice.

After helping her beloved dog Hayley transition into the Afterlife in 2007, in the comfort of home, she was guided to create Hayley's Angels Veterinary Services, the first in-home euthanasia service and end-of-life care and guidance for pets in Southern Arizona. She felt this was Hayley's legacy. Dr. Joanne has since helped over ten thousand families find peace and closure in regards to their pets' illness and passing.

With her husband, she rescues many animals of all kinds, lives as simply and sustainably as possible, and has held seven Compassionfest events over the years to promote "Caring for ALL animals, humans & our planet" in both the USA and Canada. She currently lives in Florida, USA.

She touches and opens people's hearts, she brings them back to their own essence by reconnecting with the Source, she awakens their dormant powers & passions to fulfill their life mission and live a meaningful and harmonious life. She dreams of everyone being kind and gently walking the Earth with peace, care & compassion. Her vision is to redefine our society to create a new and better normal for all animals, humans & our planet.

She hand-makes memorial charms and jewelry with a lock of hair, picture or cremains from a departed loved one to bring strength and comfort to grieving families.

Dr. Joanne is an experienced public speaker and gives lectures and workshops to promote better living and better dying with dignity for all animals and people; intuitive medicine for the mind, body and soul; living a conscious and compassionate life in balance and harmony with our world as Oneness; bridging the gap between animal owners and veterinarians by building a great team based on trust, value and loyalty; opening the heart of the beautiful medical profession by promoting compassion and communication for happier veterinarians and human doctors, happier patients and happier families; healing our health care system.

Dr. Joanne authored the book "Animal Teachings from Hayley's Angels Methods" in 2011. She is continuing to share the wisdom from animals in her second book with mind-expanding and mind-exploding animal teachings to build a better, healthier, more balanced and sustainable society to survive on our beautiful planet. She believes that animals can save us if we follow their guidance. They dare us to venture on many unexplored and controversial paths in order to discover their rich teachings!

Made in the USA
Monee, IL
08 November 2026

67380517R10100